Prostate Cancer - Latest Research Reports

Edited by Jonathan D. Kantrowitz

Published by Tsadek Press

Copyright Jonathan Kantrowitz 2014

Table of Contents

Introduction	5
Avoiding Prostate Cancer	20
Increased Prostate Cancer Risk	33
Screening for Prostate Cancer	38
Watchful Waiting	68
Chemotherapy	80
Gene Therapy	91
Hormone Therapy	95
Supplemental Therapies	
Aspirin	107
Coffee	110
Statins	117
Diet and Exercise	125
Radiation	140
Surgery	155
Prostate Cancer Survivorship	175
Last Minute Additions – Latest Research	179
Appendix- Bladder Cancer	
Increased Risk Of Bladder Cancer	187
Fighting Bladder Cancer	196
Treatment For Bladder Cancer	201

Introduction

What is Prostate Cancer?

How Tumors Form

The body is made up of many types of cells. Normally, cells grow, divide, and produce more cells as needed to keep the body healthy and functioning properly. Sometimes, however, the process goes wrong -- cells become abnormal and form more cells in an uncontrolled way. These extra cells form a mass of tissue, called a growth or tumor. Tumors can be benign, which means not cancerous, or malignant, which means cancerous.

How Prostate Cancer Occurs

Prostate cancer occurs when a tumor forms in the tissue of the prostate, a gland in the male reproductive system. In its early stage, prostate cancer needs the male hormone testosterone to grow and survive.

The prostate is about the size of a large walnut. It is located below the bladder and in front of the rectum. The prostate's main function is to make fluid for semen, a white substance that carries sperm.

Prostate cancer is one of the most common types of cancer among American men. It is a slow-growing disease that mostly affects older men. In fact, more than 60 percent of all prostate cancers are found in men over the age of 65. The disease rarely occurs in men younger than 40 years of age.

Prostate Cancer Can Spread

Sometimes, cancer cells break away from a malignant tumor in the prostate and enter the bloodstream or the lymphatic system and travel to other organs in the body.

When cancer spreads from its original location in the prostate to another part of the body such as the bone, it is called metastatic prostate cancer -- not bone cancer. Doctors sometimes call this distant disease.

Surviving Prostate Cancer

Today, more men are surviving prostate cancer than ever before. Treatment can be effective, especially when the cancer has not spread beyond the region of the prostate.

Symptoms and Tests

Symptoms

Most cancers in their early, most treatable stages don't cause any symptoms. Early prostate cancer usually does not cause symptoms.

However, if prostate cancer develops and is not treated, it can cause these symptoms:

- a need to urinate frequently, especially at night
- difficulty starting urination or holding back urine
- inability to urinate
- weak or interrupted flow of urine
- painful or burning urination
- difficulty in having an erection
- painful ejaculation
- blood in urine or semen
- pain or stiffness in the lower back, hips, or upper thighs.

Any of these symptoms may be caused by cancer, but more often they are due to enlargement of the prostate, which is not cancer.

If You Have Symptoms

If you have any of these symptoms, see your doctor or a urologist to find out if you need treatment. A urologist is a doctor who specializes in treating diseases of the genitourinary system. The doctor will ask questions about your medical history and perform an exam to try to find the cause of the prostate problems.

The PSA Test

The doctor may also suggest a blood test to check your prostate specific antigen, or PSA, level. PSA levels can be high not only in men who have prostate cancer, but also in men with an enlarged prostate gland and men with infections of the prostate. PSA tests may be very useful for early cancer diagnosis. However, PSA tests alone do not always tell whether or not cancer is present.

PSA screening for prostate cancer is not perfect. (Screening tests check for disease in a person who shows no symptoms.) Most men with mildly elevated PSA do not have prostate cancer, and many men with prostate cancer have normal levels of PSA. A recent study revealed that men with low prostate specific antigen levels, or PSA, may still have prostate cancer. Also, the digital rectal exam can miss many prostate cancers.

Other Tests

The doctor may order other exams, including ultrasound, MRI, or CT scans, to learn more about the cause of the symptoms. But to confirm the presence of cancer, doctors must perform a biopsy. During a biopsy, the doctor uses needles to remove small tissue samples from the prostate and then looks at the samples under a microscope.

If Cancer is Present

If a biopsy shows that cancer is present, the doctor will report on the grade of the tumor. Doctors describe a tumor as low, medium, or high-grade cancer, based on the way it appears under the microscope.

One way of grading prostate cancer, called the Gleason system, uses scores of 2 to 10. Another system uses G1 through G4. The higher the score, the higher the grade of the tumor. High-grade tumors grow more quickly and are more likely to spread than low-grade tumors.

Latest Research

Scientists continue to look at new ways to prevent, treat, and diagnose prostate cancer. Research has already led to a number of advances in these areas.

Dietary Research

Several studies are under way to explore the causes of prostate cancer. Some researchers think that diet may affect a man's chances of developing prostate cancer. For example, some studies show that prostate cancer is more common in populations that consume a high-fat diet, particularly animal fat, and in populations with diets that lack certain nutrients.

Research on Testosterone

Some research suggests that high levels of testosterone may increase a man's risk of prostate cancer. The difference in prostate cancer risk among racial groups could be related to high testosterone levels, but it also could result from diet or other lifestyle factors.

Genetic Research

Researchers are studying changes in genes that may increase the risk for developing prostate cancer. Some studies are looking at the genes of men who were diagnosed with prostate cancer at a relatively young age, such as less than 55 years old, and the genes of families who have several members with the disease. Other studies are trying to identify which genes, or arrangements of genes, are most likely to lead to prostate cancer. Much more work is needed, however, before scientists can say exactly how genetic changes relate to prostate cancer.

Prevention Research

Several studies have explored ways to prevent prostate cancer. In October 2008, initial results of a study on the use of the dietary supplements vitamin E and selenium found that they did not provide any benefit in reducing the number of new cases of the disease. A few studies suggest that a diet that regularly includes tomato-based foods may help protect men from prostate cancer, but there are no studies that conclusively prove this hypothesis.

According to results of a study that was re-analyzed in 2013, men who took finasteride, a drug that affects male hormone levels, reduced their chances of getting prostate cancer by nearly 30 percent compared to men who took a placebo. Unlike earlier findings from this study, this new analysis showed no increased risk of late stage disease due to use of finasteride.

Stopping Prostate Cancer from Returning

Scientists are also looking at ways to stop prostate cancer from returning in men who have already been treated for the disease. These approaches use drugs such as finasteride, flutamide, nilutamide, and LH-RH agonists that manipulate hormone levels. In 2010, the FDA approved a therapeutic cancer vaccine, Provenge, for use in some men with metastatic prostate cancer. Provenge may provide a 4-month improvement in overall survival compared with a placebo vaccine. Other similar vaccine therapies are in development.

Research on New Blood Tests

Some researchers are working to develop new blood tests to detect the antibodies that the immune system produces to fight prostate cancer. When used along with PSA testing, the antibody tests may provide more accurate results about whether or not a man has prostate cancer.

Researching New Approaches to Treatment \

Through research, doctors are trying to find new, more effective ways to treat prostate cancer. Cryosurgery -- destroying cancer by freezing it -- is under study as an alternative to surgery and radiation therapy. To avoid damaging healthy tissue, the doctor places an instrument known as a cryoprobe in direct contact with the tumor to freeze it.

Doctors are studying new ways of using radiation therapy and hormonal therapy, too. Studies have shown that hormonal therapy given after radiation therapy can help certain men whose cancer has spread to nearby tissues.

Scientists are also testing the effectiveness of chemotherapy and biological therapy for men whose cancer does not respond, or stops responding, to hormonal therapy. They are also exploring new ways to schedule and combine various treatments. For example, they are studying hormonal therapy to find out if using it to shrink the tumor before a man has surgery or radiation might be a useful approach.

For men with early stage prostate cancer, researchers are also comparing treatment with watchful waiting. The results of this work will help doctors know whether to treat early stage prostate cancer immediately or only later on, if symptoms occur or worsen.

Treatments

Choosing Treatment

There are a number of ways to treat prostate cancer, and the doctor will develop a treatment to fit each man's needs. The choice of treatment mostly depends on the stage of the disease and the grade of the tumor. But doctors also consider a man's age, general health, and his feelings about the treatments and their possible side effects.

Treatment for prostate cancer may involve watchful waiting, surgery, radiation therapy, or hormonal therapy. Some men receive a combination of therapies. A cure is the goal for men whose prostate cancer is diagnosed early.

Weighing Treatment Options

You and your doctor will want to consider both the benefits and possible side effects of each option, especially the effects on sexual activity and urination, and other concerns about quality of life.

Surgery, radiation therapy, and hormonal therapy all have the potential to disrupt sexual desire or performance for a short while or permanently. Discuss your concerns with your health care provider. Several options are available to help you manage sexual problems related to prostate cancer treatment.

Watchful Waiting

The doctor may suggest watchful waiting for some men who have prostate cancer that is found at an early stage and appears to be growing slowly. Also, watchful waiting may be advised for older men or men with other serious medical problems.

For these men, the risks and possible side effects of surgery, radiation therapy, or hormonal therapy may outweigh the possible benefits. Doctors monitor these patients with regular check-ups. If symptoms appear or get worse, the doctor may recommend active treatment.

Surgery

Surgery is used to remove the cancer. It is a common treatment for early stage prostate cancer. The surgeon may remove the entire prostate with a type of surgery called radical prostatectomy or, in some cases, remove only part of it.

Sometimes the surgeon will also remove nearby lymph nodes. Side effects of the operation may include lack of sexual function or impotence, or problems holding urine or incontinence.

Improvements in surgery now make it possible for some men to keep their sexual function. In some cases, doctors can use a technique known as nerve-sparing surgery. This may save the nerves that control erection. However, men with large tumors or tumors that are very close to the nerves may not be able to have this surgery.

Some men with trouble holding urine may regain control within several weeks of surgery. Others continue to have problems that require them to wear a pad.

Radiation Therapy

Radiation therapy uses high-energy x-rays to kill cancer cells and shrink tumors. Doctors may recommend it instead of surgery, or after surgery, to destroy any cancer cells that may remain in the area.

In advanced stages, the doctor may recommend radiation to relieve pain or other symptoms. It may also be used in combination with hormonal therapy. Radiation can cause problems with impotence and bowel function.

The radiation may come from a machine, which is external radiation, or from tiny radioactive seeds placed inside or near the tumor, which is internal radiation. Men who receive only the radioactive seeds usually have small tumors. Some men receive both kinds of radiation therapy.

For external radiation therapy, patients go to the hospital or clinic -- usually for several weeks. Internal radiation may require patients to stay in the hospital for a short time.

Hormonal Therapy

Hormonal therapy deprives cancer cells of the male hormones they need to grow and survive. This treatment is often used for prostate cancer that has spread to other parts of the body.

Sometimes doctors use hormonal therapy to try to keep the cancer from coming back after surgery or radiation treatment. Side effects can include impotence, hot flashes, loss of sexual desire, and thinning of bones. Some hormone therapies increase the risk of blood clots.

Monitoring Treatment

Regardless of the type of treatment you receive, you will be closely monitored to see how well the treatment is working. Monitoring may include

- a PSA blood test -- usually every 3 months to 1 year.

- bone scan and/or CT scan to see if the cancer has spread.

- a complete blood count to monitor for signs and symptoms of anemia.

- looking for signs or symptoms that the disease might be progressing, such as fatigue, increased pain, or decreased bowel and bladder function.

Prostate Cancer: New tests and methods take on the most commonly diagnosed cancer in men

Prostate cancer is the most commonly diagnosed cancer in males, with about 240,000 diagnoses expected this year. And there are 2.5 million people currently living with this disease. Recently there have been some dramatic changes in the way prostate cancer is diagnosed and treated. Wayne Waltzer, MD, Chairman, Department of Urology, Stony Brook Medicine explains these major medical advances and what they mean for men across the nation.

"With prostate cancer being the number one solid organ cancers in the country, it is important for all men to be vigilant about getting screened," says Dr. Waltzer. "And a newly developed series of genetic tests is now offering a more accurate and individualized approach in identifying and treating prostate cancer."

Currently there are various blood tests in use. One is called the Prostate Health Index (PHI) and the other is called the 4K test. Both measure the variance of the PSA in the blood and are designed to reduce the number of unnecessary negative biopsies that detect only low-grade cancer. "This means that not all men with elevated PSA levels will require a biopsy, with its potential for complications and side effects," says Dr. Waltzer.

There are also new tests available that help to further individualize biopsies, if one is required. "If the biopsy is positive for cancer, two tests — the Polaris and the Genomic Prostate Score — help doctors distinguish between aggressive cancers that need treatment and those that are slow growing and may need only the "watch and wait" approach," says Dr. Waltzer. "These tests work by measuring a series of genomic patterns to reveal how the cancer cells are wired to behave."

If the biopsy is negative but you still have elevated PSA levels, there is now a test called Confirm MDX that helps ensure that cancer cells were not missed during the biopsy. "The biopsy may have sampled tissue that was in an area where there were no cancer cells," says Dr. Waltzer. "This could give you a false negative. This new test looks for hyper methylation, which indicates the presence of individual prostate cancer tissue near the site of the biopsy."

If no hyper methylation is detected, the biopsy is considered negative. If some is detected, additional testing will be needed. Another test, the PCA3 test is also available in case of negative biopsy. This gene-based urine test offers additional information on the probability of finding prostate cancer in the biopsy.

In addition, if you have had prostate cancer surgery, there are genetic tests post-surgery that help determine whether additional treatment is needed based on the genetic composition of the cancer cells and the risks associated with it.

"These new tests, which are available at Stony Brook Medicine, are absolutely the future for cancer diagnostics — and not just for prostate cancer," says Dr. Waltzer. "These innovations are happening for almost every form of cancer, with more on the horizon."

Dr. Waltzer says, gene analysis of tissue, the study of genetic markers, patterns, sequencing and abnormalities, is providing physicians with unprecedented information on who to treat and how to treat them. "Not only is it helping us to find the most appropriate approach and treatment for people with cancer, but it also keeping many people with the less aggressive forms of the disease from undergoing the rigors of treatment unnecessarily. This is both a health issue and a quality of life issue. The fact that we can take such a highly individualized approach for very specific forms of cancer also means that we can look forward to better and more predictable outcomes."

Avoiding Prostate Cancer

Circumcision linked to reduced risk of prostate cancer in some men

Circumcision is performed for various reasons, including those that are based on religion, aesthetics, or health. New research indicates that the procedure may help prevent prostate cancer in some men. The findings, which are published in *BJU International*, add to a growing list of advantages to circumcision.

Besides advanced age, African ancestry, and family history of prostate cancer, no other risk factors for prostate cancer have been definitively established. This has fuelled the search for modifiable risk factors. Marie-Élise Parent, PhD and Andrea Spence, PhD, of the University of Quebec's INRS-Institut Armand-Frappier, led a team that designed an observational study to investigate the possible association between circumcision and prostate cancer risk. Their study, called PROtEuS (Prostate Cancer and Environment Study), included 1590 prostate cancer patients diagnosed in a Montréal hospital between 2005 and 2009, as well as 1618 healthy control individuals. In-person interviews were conducted to gather information on sociodemographic, lifestyle, and environmental factors.

Circumcised men had a slightly lower risk, albeit not statistically significant, of developing prostate cancer than uncircumcised men. Circumcision was found to be protective in men circumcised when they were older than 35 years, with the procedure decreasing their risk by 45%. A weaker protective effect was seen among men circumcised within 1 year of birth, with the procedure decreasing their risk by 14%. The strongest protective effect of circumcision was recorded in Black men, who had a 60% reduced risk if they were circumcised, but no association was found with other ancestral groups. "This is a particularly interesting finding, as Black men have the highest rates of prostate cancer in the world and this has never been explained," said Dr. Parent. "This novel finding warrants further examination in future studies that have a larger number of Black participants."

Dr. Parent noted that circumcision may reduce the risk of contracting and maintaining a sexually transmitted infection, which has been postulated to be a risk factor for prostate cancer. This may explain the reduced risk of prostate cancer observed in males circumcised at a younger age prior to any potential exposure to infection. "We do not know why a protective effect was observed for men circumcised after the age of 35. These men may have had a pathologic condition of the foreskin that lead to them being circumcised," she said.

Flavonoids in Fruit, and Veggies Might Fight Prostate Cancer

Prostate cancer patients who, before their diagnosis, routinely consumed hefty helpings of the flavonoid compounds found in plant-based foods and drinks may be at lower risk for the most aggressive form of the disease, new research suggests.

But the research has significant limitations, the study authors noted, so it's too soon to say that a plant-based diet protects against prostate cancer.

Flavonoids are found in vegetables and fruits, as well as in tea, wine, juices and cocoa. Researchers have long theorized that these particular antioxidants may help reduce cancer risk by fighting inflammation, oxidation, cell death and tumor cell growth.

The new study did not assess the ability of flavonoids to prevent the onset of cancer as a whole. But the investigation, involving about 1,900 patients newly diagnosed with prostate cancer, found that those whose diets included the highest amount of flavonoids were 25 percent less likely to have been diagnosed with the fastest-moving and harshest form of the disease compared to those who had been taking in the fewest flavonoids.

"We compared men with low-aggressive disease to high aggressive," said study lead author Susan Steck, associate professor at the University of South Carolina's Arnold School of Public Health. "We did not have a healthy comparison group. So while we think that consuming more fruits and vegetables will improve the odds of not getting prostate cancer altogether, we can't say that based on our study results."

"But what we are seeing here is the impact of flavonoids on reducing the risk for aggressive prostate cancer," she added. "They may not affect your risk for getting the cancer, but it may mitigate against the kind of cancer you would get."

The authors looked at self-reported dietary habits already in place at the time of diagnosis among their patient pool, which included 920 black men and 977 white men. No dietary intervention was imposed after diagnosis.

All the men had been enrolled in the North Carolina-Louisiana Prostate Cancer Project.

The new study found that smokers and men younger than 65 appeared to receive the most protective benefit from fruit and vegetable consumption.

The authors identified green and black tea, as well as orange and grapefruit juice, as the prime sources of flavonoids consumed by study participants. Strawberries, onions, cooked greens, kale and broccoli also were popular flavonoid-rich foods.

No single class of plant-based food was linked on its own to the observed protective effect, leading the team to conclude that the benefit was rooted in a dietary mix of flavonoids.

Dr. Lionel Banez, assistant professor of urologic surgery at Duke University Medical Center in Durham, N.C., said the study design makes it hard to read much into the findings.

It is "difficult to be confident about the conclusions," he said, given that the current study was a backward look at patients' recollections of their pre-diagnosis diets.

Banez suggested that the findings of a flavonoid benefit would be more reliable if they had stemmed from a highly controlled study of risk levels among patients who were proactively placed on a specific dietary plan, and then tracked for the future onset of cancer.

"These results are not enough to warrant recommending plant-based diets as regimens to treat prostate cancer or prevent aggressive prostate cancer," he said.

Although the study found an association between flavonoids and risk for a form of prostate cancer, it did not prove a cause-and-effect relationship. Because the study was presented at a medical meeting, the data and conclusions should be viewed as preliminary until published in a peer-reviewed journal.

Low Cholesterol=Lower Prostate Cancer Risk

Men with lower cholesterol are less likely than those with higher levels to develop high-grade prostate cancer - an aggressive form of the disease with a poorer prognosis, according to results of a Johns Hopkins collaborative study. In a prospective study of more than

5,000 U.S. men, epidemiologists say they now have evidence that having lower levels of heart-clogging fat may cut a man's risk of this form of cancer by nearly 60 percent.

"For many reasons, we know that it's good to have a cholesterol level within the normal range," says Elizabeth Platz, Sc.D., M.P.H., associate professor at the Johns Hopkins Bloomberg School of Public Health and co-director of the cancer prevention and control program at the Johns Hopkins Kimmel Cancer Center. "Now, we have more evidence that among the benefits of low cholesterol may be a lower risk for potentially deadly prostate cancers."

Normal range is defined as less than 200 mg/dL (milligrams per deciliter of blood) of total cholesterol.

Platz and her colleagues found similar results in a study first published in 2008, and in 2006, she linked use of cholesterol-lowering statin drugs to lower risk of advanced prostate cancer.

For the current study, Platz, members of the Southwest Oncology Group, and other collaborators analyzed data from 5,586 men aged 55 and older enrolled in the Prostate Cancer Prevention Trial from 1993 to 1996. Some 1,251 men were diagnosed with prostate cancer during the study period.

Men with cholesterol levels lower than 200 mg/dL had a 59 percent lower risk of developing high-grade prostate cancers, which tend to grow and spread rapidly. High-grade cancers are identified by a pathological ranking called the Gleason score. Scores at the highest end of the scale, between eight and 10, indicate cancers considered the most worrisome to pathologists who examine samples of the diseased prostate under the microscope.

In Platz's study, cholesterol levels had no significant effect on the entire spectrum of prostate cancer incidence, only those that were high-grade, she says.

Platz cautions that, while the group took into account factors that could bias the results, such as smoking history, weight, family history of prostate cancer, and dietary cholesterol, other things could have affected their results. One example is whether men in the study were taking cholesterol-lowering drugs at the time of the blood collections, a data point the researchers expect to analyze soon.

Results of the current study are expected to be published online Nov. 3 2009 in the journal *Cancer Epidemiology, Biomarkers & Prevention.* Also in the journal is an accompanying paper from the National Cancer Institute showing that lower cholesterol in men conferred a 15 percent decrease in overall cancer cases.

"Cholesterol may affect cancer cells at a level where it influences key signaling pathways controlling cell survival," says Platz. "Cancer cells use these survival pathways to evade the normal cycle of cell life and death."

Study confirms link between omega-3 fatty acids and increased prostate cancer risk

A second large, prospective study by scientists at Fred Hutchinson Cancer Research Center has confirmed the link between high blood concentrations of omega-3 fatty acids and an increased risk of prostate cancer.

Published in the *Journal of the National Cancer Institute,* the latest findings indicate that high concentrations of EPA, DPA and DHA – the three anti-inflammatory and metabolically related fatty acids derived from fatty fish and fish-oil supplements – are associated with a 71 percent increased risk of high-grade prostate cancer. The study also found a 44 percent increase in the risk of low-grade prostate cancer and an overall 43 percent increase in risk for all prostate cancers.

The increase in risk for high-grade prostate cancer is important because those tumors are more likely to be fatal.

The findings confirm a 2011 study published by the same Fred Hutch scientific team that reported a similar link between high blood concentrations of DHA and a more than doubling of the risk for developing high-grade prostate cancer. The latest study also confirms results from a large European study.

"The consistency of these findings suggests that these fatty acids are involved in prostate tumorigenesis and recommendations to increase long-chain omega-3 fatty acid intake, in particular through supplementation, should consider its potential risks," the authors wrote.

"We've shown once again that use of nutritional supplements may be harmful," said Alan Kristal, Dr.P.H., the paper's senior author and member of the Fred Hutch Public Health Sciences Division. Kristal also noted a recent analysis published in the Journal of the American Medical Association that questioned the benefit of omega-3 supplementation for cardiovascular diseases. The analysis, which combined the data from 20 studies, found no reduction in all-cause mortality, heart attacks or strokes.

"What's important is that we have been able to replicate our findings from 2011 and we have confirmed that marine omega-3 fatty acids play a role in prostate cancer occurrence," said corresponding author Theodore Brasky, Ph.D., a research assistant professor at The Ohio State University Comprehensive Cancer Center who was a postdoctoral trainee at Fred Hutch when the research was conducted. "It's important to note, however, that these results do not address the question of whether omega-3's play a detrimental role in prostate cancer prognosis," he said.

Kristal said the findings in both Fred Hutch studies were surprising because omega-3 fatty acids are believed to have a host of positive health effects based on their anti-inflammatory properties. Inflammation plays a role in the development and growth of many cancers.

It is unclear from this study why high levels of omega-3 fatty acids would increase prostate cancer risk, according to the authors, however the replication of this finding in two large studies indicates the need for further research into possible mechanisms. One potentially harmful effect of omega-3 fatty acids is their conversion into compounds that can cause damage to cells and DNA, and their role in immunosuppression. Whether these effects impact cancer risk is not known.

The difference in blood concentrations of omega-3 fatty acids between the lowest and highest risk groups was about 2.5 percentage points (3.2 percent vs. 5.7 percent), which is somewhat larger than the effect of eating salmon twice a week, Kristal said.

The current study analyzed data and specimens collected from men who participated in the Selenium and Vitamin E Cancer Prevention Trial (SELECT), a large randomized, placebo-controlled trial to test whether selenium and vitamin E, either alone or combined, reduced prostate cancer risk. That study showed no benefit from selenium intake and an increase in prostate cancers in men who took vitamin E.

Myths About Avoiding Prostate Cancer

When it comes to prostate cancer, there's a lot of confusion about how to prevent it, find it early and the best way -- or even whether -- to treat it. Below are four common prostate cancer myths along with research-based information from scientists at Fred Hutchinson Cancer Research Center to help men separate fact from fiction.

Myth 1 -- Eating tomato-based products such as ketchup and red pasta sauce prevents prostate cancer. "The vast majority of studies show no association," said Alan Kristal, Dr.Ph., associate director of the Hutchinson Center's Cancer Prevention Program and a national expert in prostate cancer prevention. Kristal and colleagues last year published results of the largest study to date that aimed to determine whether foods that contain lycopene -- the nutrient that puts the red in tomatoes -- actually protect against prostate cancer.

After examining blood levels of lycopene in nearly 3,500 men nationwide they found no association. "Scientists and the public should understand that early studies supporting an association of dietary lycopene with reduced prostate cancer risk have not been replicated in studies using serum biomarkers of lycopene intake," the authors reported in *Cancer Epidemiology, Biomarkers & Prevention*. "Recommendations of professional societies to the public should be modified to reflect the likelihood that increasing lycopene intake will not affect prostate cancer risk."

Myth 2 -- High testosterone levels increase the risk of prostate cancer. "This is a lovely hypothesis based on a very simplistic understanding of testosterone metabolism and its effect on prostate cancer. It is simply wrong," Kristal said. Unlike estrogen and breast cancer, where there is a very strong relationship, testosterone levels have no association with prostate cancer risk, he said. A study published in 2008 in the *Journal of the National Cancer Institute, which* combined data from 18 large studies, found no association between blood testosterone concentration and prostate cancer risk, and more recent studies have confirmed this conclusion.

Myth 3 -- Fish oil (omega-3 fatty acids) decrease prostate cancer risk. "This sounds reasonable, based on an association of inflammation with prostate cancer and the anti-inflammatory effects of omega-3 fatty acids," Kristal said. However, two large, well-designed studies -- including one led by Kristal that was published in the *American Journal of Epidemiology* -- have shown that high blood levels of omega-3 fatty acids increase the odds of developing high-risk prostate cancer.

Analyzing data from a nationwide study of nearly 3,500 men, they found that those with the highest blood percentages of docosahexaenoic acid, or DHA, an inflammation-lowering omega-3 fatty acid commonly found in fatty fish, have two-and-a-half times the risk of developing aggressive, high-grade prostate cancer compared to men with the lowest DHA levels. "This very sobering finding suggests that our understanding of the effects of omega-3 fatty acids is incomplete," Kristal said.

Myth 4 -- Dietary supplements can prevent prostate cancer. Several large, randomized trials that have looked at the impact of dietary supplements on the risk of various cancers, including prostate, have shown either no effect or, much more troubling, they have shown significantly increased risk. "The more we look at the effects of taking supplements, the more hazardous they appear when it comes to cancer risk," Kristal said. For example, the Selenium and Vitamin E Cancer Prevention Trial (SELECT), the largest prostate cancer prevention study to date, was stopped early because it found neither selenium nor vitamin E supplements alone or combined reduced the risk of prostate cancer. A SELECT follow-up study published last year in JAMA found that vitamin E actually increased the risk of prostate cancer among healthy men. The Hutchinson Center oversaw statistical analysis for the study, which involved nearly 35,000 men in the U.S., Canada and Puerto Rico.

Increased Prostate Cancer Risk

Vitamin D deficiency linked to aggressive prostate cancer

African-American and European-American men at high risk of prostate cancer have greater odds of being diagnosed with an aggressive form of the disease if they have a vitamin D deficiency, according to a new study from Northwestern Medicine® and the University of Illinois at Chicago (UIC).

Results of the study were published May 1, 2014 in *Clinical Cancer Research*, a journal of the American Association for Cancer Research.

"Vitamin D deficiency could be a biomarker of advanced prostate tumor progression in large segments of the general population," said Adam B. Murphy, M.D., lead author of the study. "More research is needed, but it would be wise for men to be screened for vitamin D deficiency and treated."

Murphy is an assistant professor in urology at Northwestern University Feinberg School of Medicine, a physician at Jesse Brown VA Medical Center and a member of the Robert H. Lurie Comprehensive Cancer Center of Northwestern University.

"This is the first study to look at vitamin D deficiency and biopsy outcomes in men at high risk of prostate cancer," said Rick Kittles, senior author of the study.

"Previous studies focused on vitamin D levels in men either with or without prostate cancer."

Kittles is an associate professor in the department of medicine at UIC.

Scientists examined data collected from a diverse group of more than 600 men from the Chicago area who had elevated PSA levels or other risk factors for prostate cancer. Each man was screened for vitamin D deficiency before undergoing a prostate biopsy.

The authors were surprised to find that vitamin D deficiency seemed to be a predictor of aggressive forms of prostate cancer diagnosis in African-American and European-American men, even after adjusting for potential confounders including diet, smoking habits, obesity, family history and calcium intake.

"These men, with severe vitamin D deficiency, had greater odds of advanced grade and advanced stage of tumors within or outside the prostate," Murphy said.

European-American men and African-American men had 3.66 times and 4.89 times increased odds of having aggressive prostate cancer respectively and 2.42 times and 4.22 times increased odds of having tumor stage T2b or higher, respectively.

African-American men with severe vitamin D deficiency also had 2.43 times increased odds of being diagnosed with prostate cancer.

"Vitamin D deficiency is more common and severe in people with darker skin and it could be that this deficiency is a contributor to prostate cancer progression among African-Americans," Murphy said. "Our findings imply that vitamin D deficiency is a bigger contributor to African-American prostate cancer."

Unless it is severe, vitamin D deficiency is fairly asymptomatic, so more effort needs to be put on screening, Murphy said.

"It is a good idea to get your levels checked on a yearly basis," Murphy said. "If you are deficient, you and you doctor can make a plan on how to reverse it through diet, supplements or other therapies."

Eating deep-fried food = increased risk of prostate cancer

Frequent, regular consumption has strongest effect and is linked to more aggressive disease

Regular consumption of deep-fried foods such as French fries, fried chicken and doughnuts is associated with an increased risk of prostate cancer, and the effect appears to be slightly stronger with regard to more aggressive forms of the disease, according to a study by investigators at Fred Hutchinson Cancer Research Center.

Corresponding author Janet L. Stanford, Ph.D., and colleagues Marni Stott-Miller, Ph.D., a postdoctoral research fellow and Marian Neuhouser, Ph.D., all of the Hutchinson Center's Public Health Sciences Division, have published their findings online in *The Prostate.*

While previous studies have suggested that eating foods made with high-heat cooking methods, such as grilled meats, may increase the risk of prostate cancer, this is the first study to examine the addition of deep frying to the equation.

Specifically, Stanford, co-director of the Hutchinson Center's Program in Prostate Cancer Research, and colleagues found that men who reported eating French fries, fried chicken, fried fish and/or doughnuts at least once a week were at an increased risk of prostate cancer as compared to men who said they ate such foods less than once a month.

In particular, men who ate one or more of these foods at least weekly had an increased risk of prostate cancer that ranged from 30 to 37 percent. Weekly consumption of these foods was associated also with a slightly greater risk of more aggressive prostate cancer. The researchers controlled for factors such as age, race, family history of prostate cancer, body-mass index and PSA screening history when calculating the association between eating deep-fried foods and prostate cancer risk.

"The link between prostate cancer and select deep-fried foods appeared to be limited to the highest level of consumption – defined in our study as more than once a week – which suggests that regular consumption of deep-fried foods confers particular risk for developing prostate cancer," Stanford said.

Screening for Prostate Cancer

New Study Questions Prostate Cancer Screening for Older Men

Only one-third of men over age 65 who receive an abnormal result from their PSA test actually undergo prostate biopsy to look for disease, a new study finds.

Prostate-specific antigen (PSA) screening is a common test that measures the level of a key marker for prostate cancer in the blood. In general, the higher the level of this protein, the more likely it is that a man has prostate cancer, according to the U.S. National Cancer Institute.

The value of the PSA test has recently come into question, however, with several studies suggesting it causes men more harm than good -- spotting too many slow-growing tumors that, especially in older patients, may never lead to serious illness or death.

The new study focused on this issue once again, tracking outcomes for nearly 300,000 men, aged 65 and older, who underwent PSA screening in the U.S. Veterans Affairs health care system in 2003. The men's health was followed for up to five years.

There were more than 25,000 men with clinically abnormal PSA levels. According to the study authors, during the five-year follow-up period, only 33 percent of those men underwent at least one prostate biopsy to check for evidence of cancer. About 63 percent of those who did have a biopsy were diagnosed with prostate cancer, of whom 82 percent were treated for their cancer.

The older the man, the less likely he was to have a prostate biopsy after having an abnormal PSA screening test result. Men with other health problems were also less likely to undergo a prostate biopsy, the investigators reported.

The study was published in the journal *JAMA Internal Medicine*.

Among men with biopsy-detected prostate cancer, the risk of death from causes other than prostate cancer increased with age and with the presence of other health problems, Dr. Louise Walter, of San Francisco Veterans Affairs Medical Center, and colleagues pointed out in a journal news release.

Two experts not connected to the study said the findings weren't surprising, given the patients' ages.

"PSA screening has been controversial as it has a relatively low yield for finding clinically significant cancer as well as potential complications and expense related to diagnosis and treatment," said Dr. Louis Kavoussi, chairman of urology at North Shore-LIJ's Arthur Institute for Urology in New Hyde Park, N.Y.

In the new study, "as age and other chronic illnesses of aging increased, the less likely biopsy was performed," he said. "This makes sense as the authors report that older individuals and those with [other illnesses] are more likely to die of a non-prostate cancer-related cause."

Therefore, the decision to test for PSA levels in older men must take into account their relatively low risk of dying of prostate cancer, Kavoussi said. "Overall, it is known that about 10 percent of individuals diagnosed with prostate cancer succumb to the disease," he said. "In this older patient population study it was 2.2 percent -- much lower, but not zero."

Another expert agreed, saying that younger men may benefit most from regular PSA screening.

"For screening to be effective, we need to focus on men with a long life expectancy," said Dr. Stacy Loeb, assistant professor in the department of population health at NYU Langone Medical Center, New York City. "Screening allows us to diagnose the life-threatening cancers in time for cure [but] diagnosis does not mandate treatment," she explained.

"Once a diagnosis is made, many patients with low risk disease can be safely monitored conservatively," Loeb said. "Men should be actively involved in all of these choices, with a discussion about risks and benefits."

What's really needed, according to Kavoussi, is a screen that can tell a patient whether his prostate cancer is aggressive or not.

There's a "need for better ways of detecting clinically significant disease in this older population, both to avoid overtreatment and to minimize the risk of missing significant disease," Kavoussi said.

PSA Screening Benefits Few, Harms Many, Says Panel

A US government-sponsored panel of independent experts that reviews evidence and develops recommendations for preventive clinical services says the harms of PSA-based testing for prostate cancer outweigh the benefits. The recommendation has provoked a strong and angry response from many patient and medical groups.

In a report published in the *Annals of Internal Medicine*, the US Preventive Services Task Force (USPSTF) writes of PSA-based screening for prostate cancer: "[it] may benefit a small number of men but will result in harm to many others".

The USPSTF is a group of primary care physicians and epidemiologists that is appointed and funded by the US Department of Health and Human Services' Agency for Healthcare Research and Quality (AHRQ). Its recommendations are important because they influence how health policy is shaped and what insurers do. For instance, it is empowered by the Affordable Care Act to decide which screenings Americans receive.

This recommendation is the task force's "final word" on PSA-based testing. It follows a period of public comment after its last published recommendation in 2008, when at the time it concluded there was no evidence to support PSA testing for men over 75.

The task force says it has since then reviewed the evidence published since 2008 and concluded that the harms of PSA-based testing outweigh the benefits, regardless of age. The task force does not take costs into account when developing recommendations: it just weighs health benefits against harms.

The task force posted a draft of this final recommendation for public comment in October 2011. At the time it gave PSA-based screening a "D" grade, which means doctors should not offer the test to their patients because there are more harms than benefits.

Many who commented at the time suggested the "D" be changed to a "C" which says doctors could offer the test to patients who ask for it. But the panel has not changed its draft recommendation, and has stuck to the "D" grade.

According to its Annals of Internal Medicine report, the task force considered two major trials that assessed the life-saving benefits of PSA-based testing in asymptomatic men.

The first trial took place in the US. It did not show that

PSA-screening reduce deaths to prostate cancer. The second trial took place in seven European countries and found PSA screening reduced deaths by one death per 1,000 men screened in a subgroup aged 5 to 69 years, mostly in two countries. The other five countries did not find a statistically significant reduction deaths.

The task force reports there is strong evidence that PSA-based screening can be harmful.

Just under 90% of men whose prostate cancer is detected via PSA undergo early treatment, either with surgery, radiation, or androgen deprivation therapy, they write. They say the evidence shows up to 5 out of every 1,000 men die within 1 month of surgery, and between 10 and 70 that survive have to live the rest of their lives with urinary incontinence, erectile and bowel dysfunction.

Leading Experts Disagree On Evidence Behind Prostate Cancer Screening Recommendations

Do the results of recent randomized trials justify the recent U.S. recommendation against yearly measurement of prostate-specific antigen (PSA) as a screening test for prostate cancer? That's the topic of debate in a special "point/counterpoint" section in the April issue of Medical Care.

The recommendation against routine PSA measurement relies too heavily on randomized trial data, according to an article by Ruth Etzioni, PhD, of Fred Hutchinson

Cancer Research Center, Seattle, and colleagues. They argue that modeling studies provide a truer picture of the long-term benefits of PSA screening. But Dr Joy Melnikow of University of California, Davis, and colleagues disagree, asserting that randomized trials provide a sufficient level of certainty to recommend against PSA screening.

Point: Short-Term Trials Don't Reflect Long-Term Risk
Last year, the U.S. Preventive Services Task Force recommended against routine PSA measurement to screen for prostate cancer. The recommendation was mainly based on two recent studies -- one conducted in Europe and one in the United States -- in which men were randomly assigned to annual PSA screening or no screening. Both studies concluded that annual screening did not reduce the risk of death from prostate cancer.

But randomized trials have important limitations as a basis for screening policies, according to Dr Etzioni and colleagues. They note that screening trials generally provide short-term results, in contrast to the long-term results generated by population-wide screening programs. They argue that taking the randomized trial data at face value "misrepresents the likely long-term population impact of PSA screening (relative to no screening) in the United States."

Dr Etzioni and coauthors discuss the results of modeling studies that give a different picture of the benefits of PSA screening. Based on those models, screening may explain 45 percent of recent declines in U.S. deaths from prostate cancer, while changes in treatment account for 33 percent. When the randomized trial data are extrapolated to the U.S. population over the long term, the absolute reduction in deaths attributed to screening appears at least five times greater than in the original trial reports.

Modeling studies also suggest a lower rate of overdiagnosis -- screening detection of slow-growing prostate cancers that otherwise would have caused no harm -- than reported in the trials. Dr Etzioni and colleagues conclude, "With a disease whose hallmark is a lengthy natural history, the harms of developing cancer screening policies based primarily on limited-duration screening trials may well outweigh the benefits."

Counterpoint: Trials Are Best Evidence on Screening Effects But in their "Counterpoint" essay, by Dr Melnikow and colleagues notes that the U.S. and European trials provided 11 to 13 years' follow-up in more than 250,000 individuals. They also point out that the U.S. trial was highly representative of the population and showed no reduction in death resulting from annual PSA testing. (Dr Melnikow and colleagues were members of the U.S. Preventive Services Task Force when the recommendation was made.)

They add that, because of "competing causes of death," it becomes even less likely that a large reduction in deaths from prostate cancer will appear over long-term follow-up. The chances of overdiagnosis and potential harms from screening are also likely to increase with continued aging. Dr Melnikow and coauthors conclude, "Projections from models are subject to mistaken assumptions and investigator biases, and should not be accorded the same weight as evidence from randomized controlled trials."

In an editorial response, Dr Etzioni's group points out that modeling plays an essential role in addressing questions about the harms and benefits of screening. "While we acknowledge the centrality of screening trials in the policy process," they write, "we maintain that modeling constitutes a powerful tool for screening trial interpretation and screening policy development."

The debate is "no mere academic exercise," according to an editorial by Ronnie D. Horner, PhD, of University of Cincinnati Medical Center. With the increased emphasis on disease prevention under health care reform, it is essential to offer those services most likely to represent value -- including cancer screenings. While there's no easy answer, Dr Horner writes, "I am hopeful that this Point-Counterpoint exchange will initiate a discussion among healthcare scientists that will yield greater guidance for determining whether a health care service is, indeed, value health care."

PSA-testing and early treatment decreases risk of prostate cancer death

The study is based on data from nation-wide, population-based registers in Sweden including the Cancer Register,

The Cause of Death Register and the National Prostate Cancer Register (NPCR) of Sweden.

"Our results show that prostate cancer mortality was 20 procent lower in counties with the highest incidence of prostate cancer, indicating an early and rapid uptake of PSA testing, compared with counties with a slow and late increase in PSA testing," says Pär Stattin, lead investigator of the study.

"Since the difference in the number of men diagnosed with prostate cancer is related to how many men undergo PSA testing, we think our data shows that PSA testing and early treatment is related to a modest decrease in risk of prostate cancer death," says Håkan Jonsson statistician and senior author of the study.

"In contrast to screening in randomized studies our data is based on unorganized, real life PSA testing. We therefore used a statistical method that excludes men that were diagnosed prior to the introduction of PSA testing since these men could not benefit from the effect of PSA testing," continues Håkan Jonsson.

"The results in our study are very similar to those obtained in a large European randomized clinical study (ERSPC) thus confirming the effect of PSA testing on the risk of prostate cancer death. However, we have to bear in mind that the decrease in mortality is offset by overtreatment and side effects from early treatment. PSA testing sharply increases the risk of overtreatment, i.e. early treatment of cancers that would never have surfaced clinically. We also know that after surgery for prostate cancer most men have decreased erectile function and that a small group of men suffer from urinary incontinence. Our data pinpoints the need for refined methods for PSA testing and improved prostate cancer treatment strategies," concludes Dr .Stattin.

Myths About PSA Tests

When it comes to prostate cancer, there's a lot of confusion about how to find it early and the best way -- or even whether -- to treat it. Below are ftwocommon prostate cancer myths along with research-based information from scientists at Fred Hutchinson Cancer Research Center to help men separate fact from fiction.

Myth 1 -- We don't know which prostate cancers detected by PSA (prostate-specific antigen) screening need to be treated and which ones can be left alone. "Actually, we have a very good sense of which cancers have a very low risk of progression and which ones are highly likely to spread if left untreated," said biostatistician Ruth Etzioni, Ph.D., a member of the Hutchinson Center's Public Health Sciences Division.

In addition to blood levels of PSA, indicators of aggressive disease include tumor volume (the number of biopsy samples that contain cancer) and Gleason score (predicting the aggressiveness of cancer by how the biopsy samples look under a microscope). Gleason scores range from 2-5 (low risk) and 6-7 (medium risk) to 8-10 (high risk).

"Men with a low PSA level, a biopsy Gleason score of 6 or lower and very few biopsy samples with cancer are generally considered to be very low risk," Etzioni said. Such newly diagnosed men increasingly are being offered active surveillance -- a watchful waiting approach -- rather than therapy for their disease, particularly if they are older or have a short life expectancy.

"The chance that these men will die of their disease if they are not treated is very low, around 3 percent," she said. Similarly, such men who opt for treatment have a mortality rate of about 2 percent. "For the majority of newly diagnosed cases of prostate cancer, giving initial clinical and biopsy information, we can get a very good idea of who should be treated and who is likely to benefit from deferring treatment."

Myth 2 -- Only one in 50 men diagnosed with PSA screening benefits from treatment. "This number, which was released as a preliminary result from the European Randomized Study of Prostate Cancer Screening, is simply incorrect," Etzioni said. "It suggests a very unfavorable harm-benefit ratio for PSA screening. It implies that for every man whose life is saved by PSA screening, almost 50 are overdiagnosed and overtreated."

"Overdiagnosis" is diagnosing a disease that will never cause symptoms or death in the patient's lifetime.

"Overtreatment" is treating a disease that will never progress to become symptomatic or life-threatening.

The 50-to-one ratio is based on short-term follow-up and "grossly underestimates" the lives likely to be saved by screening over the long term and overestimates the number who are overdiagnosed. "The correct ratio of men diagnosed with PSA testing who are overdiagnosed and overtreated versus men whose lives are saved by treatment long term is more likely to be 10 to one," she said.

A New Screening Method for Prostate Cancer: PSA Velocity Risk Count Testing

A new study by NYU Langone Medical Center and Northwestern University Feinberg School of Medicine shows novel PSA velocity (PSAV) risk count testing may provide a more effective way for physicians to screen men for clinically significant prostate cancer. The new study, published online by the *British Journal of Urology International on* February 1, 2012, shows the benefits of tracking a man's PSA levels over time to help doctors more accurately assess his risk of life-threatening prostate cancer.

"Risk count could represent a new way to screen for prostate cancer by focusing on men with the greatest risk of harmful prostate cancers," said lead author Stacy Loeb, MD, an urologist in the Department of Urology and the Joel E. Smilow Comprehensive Prostate Cancer Center at NYU Langone. "The goal of risk count is to help identify the aggressive, clinically significant prostate cancers before advanced symptoms develop, while decreasing the diagnosis of insignificant cancers."

Prostate cancer is the second leading cause of cancer death in American men, with an estimated 1 in 6 men diagnosed with the disease during their lifetime. Prostate cancer does not present symptoms until advanced stages so screening for the disease is vital. Currently, a PSA blood test is the standard screening method to evaluate a man's risk of prostate cancer. It measures the amount of prostate-specific antigen in the blood, a substance made only in the prostate gland. An elevated PSA can indicate the presence of disease. However, PSA can also be elevated with benign prostate enlargement and one high PSA value does not always mean an aggressive prostate cancer is present.

The new PSAV risk count screening works by monitoring fluctuations in PSA levels over time to analyze a man's risk of prostate cancer, instead of relying on just one PSA test result to assign prostate cancer risk. The risk count is calculated by counting the number of times in a row that the PSA level in the blood increases by 0.4 ng/mL. If PSA goes up by more than 0.4 units multiple years in a row, the risk count rises indicating the patient has an increased risk of aggressive prostate cancer. For example, a man who has a PSA screening for two years in a row would be given a "2" risk count if his serial PSA velocity measurements increased by more than 0.4 units, a "1" risk count if there was only one increase by more than 0.4 units, and a "0" risk count if there was no increase by more than 0.4 units.

In the study, researchers showed PSAV risk count could improve the specificity of screening for prostate cancer and advanced stages of the disease. Researchers evaluated 18, 214 men undergoing prostate cancer screening, 1,125 of which were diagnosed with the disease. The study results show sustained rises in PSA levels over time indicate a significantly greater risk of prostate cancer and more aggressive disease. In the study, a risk count of "2" was associated with a greater than 8-times risk of prostate cancer and a 5-fold greater risk of aggressive disease.

The authors conclude risk count screening may be useful in diagnosing aggressive prostate cancer earlier while possibly reducing unnecessary biopsy, as well as the overdiagnosis and resulting overtreatment of low-risk prostate cancer.

"A persistently rising PSA is a harbinger for life-threatening prostate cancer," said the study's senior author, William Catalona, MD, professor of Urology at Northwestern University. "Our study findings show looking at how much PSA changes over time helps distinguish which cancers are aggressive more so than a single PSA value."

In an accompanying editorial, Dr. H. Ballentine Carter

from the Brady Urological Institute at Johns Hopkins who initially suggested the concept of looking at PSA changes over time, affirms that in order to determine the likelihood of aggressive prostate cancer, "you want to know your patient's risk count, not just their age and PSA level."

Prostate cancer biomarkers identified in seminal fluid

Improved diagnosis and management of one of the most common cancers in men – prostate cancer – could result from research at the University of Adelaide, which has discovered that seminal fluid (semen) contains biomarkers for the disease.

Results of a study now published in the journal Endocrine-Related Cancer have shown that the presence of certain molecules in seminal fluid indicates not only whether a man has prostate cancer, but also the severity of the cancer.

Speaking in the lead-up to Men's Health Week 2014, (9-15 June) University of Adelaide research fellow and lead author Dr Luke Selth says the commonly used PSA (prostate specific antigen) test is by itself not ideal to test for the cancer.

"While the PSA test is very sensitive, it is not highly specific for prostate cancer," Dr Selth says. "This results in many unnecessary biopsies of non-malignant disease.

More problematically, PSA testing has resulted in substantial over-diagnosis and over-treatment of slow growing, non-lethal prostate cancers that could have been safely left alone.

"Biomarkers that can accurately detect prostate cancer at an early stage and identify aggressive tumors are urgently needed to improve patient care. Identification of such biomarkers is a major focus of our research," he says.

Dr Selth, a Young Investigator of the Prostate Cancer Foundation (USA), is a member of the Freemasons Foundation Centre for Men's Health at the University of Adelaide and is based in the University's Dame Roma Mitchell Cancer Research Laboratories.

Using samples from 60 men, Dr Selth and colleagues discovered a number of small ribonucleic acid (RNA) molecules called microRNAs in seminal fluid that are known to be increased in prostate tumors. The study showed that some of these microRNAs were surprisingly accurate in detecting cancer.

"The presence of these microRNAs enabled us to more accurately discriminate between patients who had cancer and those who didn't, compared with a standard PSA test," Dr Selth says. "We also found that the one specific microRNA, miR-200b, could distinguish between men with low grade and higher grade tumors. This is important because, as a potential prognostic tool, it will help to indicate the urgency and type of treatment required."

This research builds on previous work by Dr Selth's team, published in the British Journal of Cancer, which demonstrated that microRNAs in the blood can predict men who are likely to relapse after surgical removal of their prostate cancer. "We are excited by the potential clinical application of microRNAs in a range of body fluids," he says.

PSA Testing, Combined With Other Relevant Patient Data Can Reduce Unnecessary Prostate Biopsies

Separate study suggests combining urine test with PSA can aid cancer diagnosis

Prostate cancer screening that combines an adjusted blood test with other factors including the size of the gland, the patient's overall weight and family history, can help up to one-quarter of men avoid biopsies and the risks associated with them, a Beth Israel Deaconess Medical Center-led research team says.

Writing in a study published online by the journal *Cancer,* the team led by Martin G. Sanda, MD, Director of the Prostate Center at Beth Israel Deaconess Medical Center and Professor of Urology at Harvard Medical School, suggests that instead of using "one-size-fits-all" levels of PSA to determine who should have a biopsy, considering other factors such as prostate size can substantially improve the ability of PSA testing to identify aggressive prostate cancers for which treatment is warranted, while avoiding detection of indolent cancers that are better undiagnosed because they do not require treatment.

A second study led by Sanda, and published online in the journal *Urologic Oncology,* suggests the presence or absence of genes commonly found in the urine of men, when combined with a PSA test, can also be used to determine whether a biopsy is necessary.
The new suggested approaches come as the United States Preventive Services Task Force expert panel concluded that current PSA-based prostate cancer screening saves few or no lives, but causes harm through treatment or further invasive testing such as biopsies. That's because prostate cancers can vary in aggressiveness and more men die of other causes aside from that cancer – and because the PSA test alone cannot determine how dangerous any particular cancer may be.

"The US Preventative Services Task Force threw the baby out with the bathwater by their blanket recommendation against prostate cancer screening," says Sanda, noting that PSA screening can instead be refined to more selectively identify only aggressive cancer for which treatment is indicated by adjusting PSA results for other considerations such as family history, obesity, and prostate size.

Results from the multi-center study that suggest that

PSAD levels of less than 0.1 – in contrast to the unadjusted level of between 2.5 and 4 – can be a better benchmark of a potential cancer. The density, determined by a digital rectal exam, enables physicians to take into account other factors like benign prostatic hyperplasia, an enlargement of the gland that affects all men as they age.

Combining the PSAD with the digital exam, a look at the patient's family history and a body mass index of 25 of less – the calculation used to define obesity – would avoid biopsy in approximately one-quarter of biopsy-eligible men, the researchers found.

"Urological practice, patient outcome and cost-effectiveness of health care would each benefit from new targeted strategies, such as nomograms (a predictive tool) that improve prediction of aggressive cancers, to enable selective identification of candidate for prostate biopsy that would improve the yield of clinically significant, histologically aggressive cancers warranting subsequent definitive treatment," researchers wrote.

In a separate multicenter study published in Urologic Oncology, researchers said a test looking for two specific genetic biomarkers – TMPRSS2:ERG and PCA3 – taken after a digital rectal exam, could help limit biopsies to men who possess both genes and whose PSA readings range between 2 and 10, potentially sparing one-third of men from biopsies.

"Urine testing for prostate cancer is in its infancy," says Sanda, noting next steps are underway as a result of study funded by a $3.1 million grant from the National Institutes of Health , that is evaluating new urine and blood test for prostate cancer in more 2,400 men over the next five years with a goal of improving upon the problems of over-diagnosis and over-treatment.

A focal point of the proposed work involves a community outreach effort led by BIDMC primary care physician J. Jacques Carter, MD, MPH, Medical Director of the Dana Farber Cancer Institute Prostate Cancer Screening and Education Program and an Assistant Professor of Medicine at Harvard Medical School. A key component of this study will be African-American men, who appear to develop prostate cancer more frequently, and who are at increased risk of dying from prostate cancer.

Age a Big Factor in Prostate Cancer Deaths

Contrary to common belief, men age 75 and older are diagnosed with late-stage and more aggressive prostate cancer and thus die from the disease more often than younger men, according to a University of Rochester analysis published online this week by the journal, Cancer.

The study is particularly relevant in light of the recent controversy about prostate cancer screening. Earlier this month a government health panel said that healthy men age 50 and older should no longer be routinely tested for prostate cancer because the screening test in its current form does not save lives and sometimes leads to needless suffering and overtreatment. Patient advocates and many clinicians disagreed with the finding.

Although the Rochester study does not address screening directly it does raise questions about the benefits of earlier detection among the elderly.

"Especially for older people, the belief is that if they are diagnosed with prostate cancer it will grow slowly and they will die of something else," said lead author Guan Wu, M.D., Ph.D., assistant professor of Urology and of Pathology and Laboratory Medicine at the University of Rochester Medical Center.

"We hope our study will raise awareness of the fact that older men are actually dying at high rates from prostate cancer," he said. "With an aging population it is important to understand this, as doctors and patients will be embarking on more discussions about the pros and cons of treatment."

Wu and colleagues studied the largest national cohort of cancer patients, called the Surveillance, Epidemiology, and End Results (SEER) database. They analyzed 464,918 records of men diagnosed with prostate cancer between 1998 and 2007, known as the "PSA era" because of a strong inclination to recommend the PSA test during that time.

(The prostate-specific antigen or PSA is a protein produced by the prostate gland, which can be measured in the blood. An elevated PSA is associated with cancer and other noncancerous prostate conditions.)

The analysis showed that when age groups are broken down into smaller sections, men 75 or older represented only 16 percent of the male population above age 50 and 26 percent of all cases of prostate cancer -- but 48 percent of cases of metastatic disease at diagnosis and 53 percent of all deaths. In general, higher grade cancer seemed to increase with age, the study said.

Researchers were looking for associations between age, metastasis and death because in clinical practice, Wu said, several URMC urologists observed that many otherwise healthy older men were presenting with very advanced disease at diagnosis, and reporting that they had never had a PSA test.

Indeed, older men have largely been excluded from prior clinical trials of the benefits of early detection, the study said. This is based on the idea that older men wouldn't benefit from early detection because of a shorter remaining life expectancy.

But Wu and colleagues contend that overall health, more than age, impacts life expectancy following a cancer diagnosis, and that more studies are needed to identify ways to manage the disease in older patients.

"Due to a lot of natural variation in the biology of prostate cancer," Wu said, "the URMC study should stimulate the need to develop an algorithm to identify healthy, elderly men who might benefit from an earlier diagnosis."

Inflammation Marker may Guide Prognosis for Prostate Cancer

Current methods of prostate cancer detection, like the prostate-specific antigen (PSA) test, often fail to identify which cancers will prove fatal and which cancers will remain benign until a patient dies of other causes.

"We are in need of better markers that distinguish between aggressive and indolent disease in this population," said Jennifer R. Rider, Sc.D., an instructor in medicine at the Brigham and Women's Hospital, Harvard Medical School in Boston, Mass.

In a study published September 2011 in *Cancer Epidemiology, Biomarkers & Prevention,* a journal of the American Association for Cancer Research, Rider and colleagues suggested that levels of prostatic intraepithelial neoplasia (PIN) could allow for a more precise prognosis.

The researchers evaluated men with localized prostate cancer diagnosed following a surgical procedure to treat benign prostatic hyperplasia. Of these men, 228 died of prostate cancer and 387 were diagnosed with prostate cancer, but were still alive after 10 years. Those with PIN were 89 percent more likely to die of prostate cancer.

Even after accounting for age, Gleason score, year of diagnosis, inflammation and type of focal atrophy present, PIN still managed to independently predict the lethality of a given tumor. There was also a suggestion that the degree of chronic inflammation adjacent to the tumor could predict lethal outcome.

"Identifying features surrounding the tumor that can predict prognosis, such as the presence of PIN or inflammation, can improve our understanding of the biology of aggressive prostate cancer and help to guide clinical decision-making," said Rider.

Change in PSA levels over time can help predict aggressive prostate cancer

Measurements taken over time of prostate specific antigen, the most commonly used screening test for prostate cancer in men, improve the accuracy of aggressive prostate cancer detection when compared to a single measurement of PSA, according to a Kaiser Permanente study published in the *British Journal of Urology International*.

The retrospective study examined the electronic health records of nearly 220,000 men ages 45 and older over a

10-year period who had at least one PSA measurement and no previous diagnosis of prostate cancer. The study found that annual percent changes in PSA more accurately predicted the presence of aggressive prostate cancer when compared to single measurements of PSA alone, but only marginally improved the prediction of prostate cancer overall.

"The use of a single, elevated PSA level to screen for prostate cancer is considered controversial given the questionable benefits of PSA screening on prostate cancer mortality. The screening may also result in unnecessary prostate biopsies and subsequent treatments for localized prostate cancer, as it does not distinguish well between slow-growing and aggressive disease," said Lauren P. Wallner, PhD, MPH, study lead author and post-doctoral research fellow at Kaiser Permanente Southern California's Department of Research & Evaluation. "Our study demonstrates that repeated measurements of PSA over time could provide a more accurate – and much needed – detection strategy for aggressive forms of prostate cancer."

Men in the study were also found to experience a 2.9 percent change in PSA levels per year on average and that the rate of change in PSA increased modestly with age.

"The results of this study could provide clinicians with a better prostate cancer preventive strategy that could help differentiate between men with an aggressive form of the disease and those who have slow-growing, indolent cancer that may not necessarily merit treatment," said Wallner. "While we do not suggest that patients proactively seek out additional PSA measurements, men who already have had multiple PSAs may consider discussing the change in their PSA levels with their clinician when determining future treatment strategies."

The PSA test measures the level of prostate specific antigen, a substance made by the prostate, in a man's blood. It is one of the most commonly used tests to screen for prostate cancer, according to the Centers for Disease Control and Prevention. As a rule, the higher the PSA level in the blood, the more likely a prostate problem is present. But many factors, such as age, race, and non-cancerous conditions can affect PSA levels. The CDC and other federal agencies follow the prostate cancer screening recommendations set forth by the U.S. Preventive Services Task Force, which recommends against PSA-based screening for men who do not have symptoms. Kaiser Permanente guidelines include a recommendation that men age 40 and older should discuss the PSA test and rectal exam with their physician.

Aside from non-melanoma skin cancer, prostate cancer is the most common cancer among men in the United States, according to the CDC. In 2008 (the most recent year numbers are available), nearly 215,000 men in the United States were diagnosed with prostate cancer and more than 28,000 men died from the disease. Prostate cancer is the second most common cause of death from cancer among white, African American, American

Indian/Alaska Native and Hispanic men, and is more common in African-American men than white men, according to the CDC.

New data shows ProMark accurately predicts aggressive prostate cancer, pathology outcomes

Metamark has presented results from the clinical validation study that showed ProMark™, the first and only proteomic-based imaging biopsy test, achieved its primary endpoint by accurately differentiating between aggressive and non-aggressive forms of prostate cancer at early stages of disease. ProMark™ was shown to predict which patients have low-risk disease with a sensitivity of 90 percent or better, confidently identifying patients who are appropriate for active surveillance or need aggressive therapy. The data was presented at the 2014 Annual Meeting of the American Society of Clinical Oncology (ASCO).

"These results reinforce ProMark™ as a critical tool that has the potential to improve prostate cancer care by fulfilling the unmet need for more precise prognostic testing, which may benefit a significant number of the more than 200,000 men in the U.S. diagnosed annually who may be appropriate for active surveillance," said Fred Saad, M.D., F.R.C.S., Professor and Chief, Division of Urology, Director of Urologic Oncology, University of Montreal Hospital Center. "ProMark™ offers the oncology healthcare community a novel prognostic option to help confidently differentiate patients with more aggressive cancers from those with less aggressive disease, thereby enabling more personalized treatment decisions for our patients."

The results being presented are a culmination of three clinical studies. The first study identified 12 biomarkers that predicted both lethal outcome and prostate cancer pathology, and of those, eight were targeted in a clinical development biopsy study as the final subset for the ProMark™ test.

The third, blinded clinical validation study of ProMark™, which analyzed 274 prostate cancer biopsies, accurately predicted the overall prostate cancer pathology for patients with biopsy Gleason grades of 3+3 (=6) or 3+4 (=7). Quantitative measurements on the biopsy samples allowed researchers to successfully identify ProMark™ risk scores for 'favorable' cases (surgical Gleason score 3+3 or 3+4; organ-confined disease [<=pT2]) as potential candidates for active surveillance and 'unfavorable' cases ($\geq$T3a, N, or M or surgical Gleason >=4+3), more likely in need of aggressive therapy, with an AUC of 0.69 (0.61-0.74; p<0.0001) and odd's ratios lowest to highest quartile of 5.

Researchers found that patients with low-risk ProMark™ scores (<0.33) were accurately identified as having favorable disease 81 percent of the time, with 90 percent specificity, while high-risk scores (>0.8) indicating non-favorable disease were predicted 77 percent of the time.

Importantly, the ProMark™ test was found to provide additional, independent prediction relative to standard risk-stratification systems, including National Comprehensive Cancer Network (NCCN) guidelines, the D'Amico system, and CAPRA, all using Prostate-Specific Antigen (PSA) levels, Gleason grades and T stage to group men as low, intermediate, or high-risk.

"A key challenge in treating men with prostate cancer is determining whether they need aggressive therapy, or if active surveillance is appropriate. Current clinical and pathological parameters are insufficient in predicting the risk of aggressive cancer for early stage cancer patients" said Peter Blume-Jensen, M.D., Ph.D., Senior Vice President and Chief Scientific Officer at Metamark. "ProMark™ was developed with the specific purpose to address this need. This latest data is a significant milestone for Metamark as it indicates ProMark™ can be used as an objective aid in decision making together with standard-of-care for prostate cancer prognosis, and thereby help maintain a higher quality of life for patients by avoiding unnecessary aggressive therapy, like surgical prostatectomy or radiation."

Watchful Waiting

Most prostate cancer specialists don't recommend active surveillance for low-risk patients

Specialists who treat prostate cancer agree that active surveillance is an effective option—yet most don't recommend it when appropriate for their own patients, according to a study in the July 2014 issue of Medical Care . The journal is published by Lippincott Williams & Wilkins , a part of Wolters Kluwer Health.

Rather, urologists are more likely to recommend surgery and radiation oncologists are more likely to recommend radiation therapy—the treatments provided by their own specialties. "Given the growing concerns about the overtreatment of prostate cancer, our study has important policy implications about possible barriers to promoting active surveillance and specialty biases about optimal treatment regarding localized prostate cancer," comments Dr Simon P. Kim of Yale School of Medicine.

Most Prostate Specialists Rate Active Surveillance Effective…

The researchers surveyed urologists and radiation oncologists regarding their views on options for "low-risk" prostate cancer. The study focused on perceptions of active surveillance as an initial approach.

Prostate cancer typically progresses slowly—most older men diagnosed with early-stage disease won't actually die of prostate cancer. For these low-risk cases, there's growing interest in active surveillance, in which patients are closely monitored for evidence of disease progression.

Active surveillance has emerged as an approach to avoid "overtreatment" of prostate cancer. In many cases, it can avoid surgery or radiation therapy that would entail a risk of complications and side effects without actually benefiting the patient.

Dr Kim and coauthors analyzed survey responses from 717 US urologists and radiation oncologists. Consistent with the research evidence, 72 percent of the specialists agreed that active surveillance is an effective alternative for men with low-risk prostate cancer. In addition, 80 percent agreed that active surveillance was underused in the United States.

…But Don't Recommend It for Their Own Patients

"However, 71 percent of the physicians responded that their patients were not interested in active surveillance," the researchers write. The rate was over 80 percent for radiation oncologists, compared to 60 percent for urologists.

When asked what treatment they would recommend for a hypothetical 60-year-old man with low-risk prostate cancer, just 22 percent of the physicians said would endorse active surveillance. Instead, 45 percent would recommend surgery (radical prostatectomy) while 35 percent would recommend some form of radiation therapy.

In general, the recommendations split along specialty lines—most respondents recommended the treatment provided by their specialty. After adjustment for other factors, urologists were four times more likely to recommend surgery, compared to radiation oncologists. Urologists were also much less likely to recommend any form of radiation therapy.

Urologists were more than twice as likely to recommend active surveillance, compared to radiation oncologists. Doctors who worked in academic medical centers were also more likely to recommend active surveillance.

The survey adds to recent evidence that physicians view active surveillance as a "reasonable approach" to initial treatment in appropriate patients with low-risk prostate cancer. Both groups of specialists acknowledge the growing concern about overtreatment of prostate cancer.

However, "that hasn't consistently translated into their self-reported patterns of treatment recommendations," Dr Kim and colleagues write. "Our study suggests that there remain some key attitudinal barriers to active surveillance among prostate cancer specialists, especially considering radiation oncologists and urologists may view their treatment as superior."

The researchers discuss some options to better incorporate patient preferences into treatment decisions—such as decision aids to provide men with evidence-based data on the advantages and disadvantages of treatment options. Coordinated, multidisciplinary care involving the patient's primary care providers as well as specialists may also provide a better balance between the risks and benefits of the different approaches. "By doing so, active surveillance may become a more acceptable disease management strategy for low-risk prostate cancer among newly diagnosed patients and specialists," Dr Kim and coauthors conclude.

Investigational urine test can predict high-risk prostate cancer in men who chose 'watchful waiting'

Initial results of a multicenter study coordinated by researchers at Fred Hutchinson Cancer Research Center indicates that two investigational urine-based biomarkers are associated with prostate cancers that are likely to be aggressive and potentially life-threatening among men who take a "watchful waiting," or active-surveillance approach to manage their disease. Ultimately, these markers may lead to the development of a urine test that could complement prostate biopsy for predicting disease aggressiveness and progression.

Study principal investigator Daniel Lin, M.D., an associate member of the Hutchinson Center's Public

Health Sciences Division, presented these findings at the 2012 Genitourinary Cancers Symposium of the American Society of Clinical Oncology in San Francisco.

"Prostate biopsies are invasive and don't always pick up all of the cancer. Post-digital-rectal exam urine collection is much less invasive. If a urine-based diagnostic test could be developed that could help predict aggressive disease or disease progression, that would be ideal," said Lin, who is also an associate professor and chief of urologic oncology at the University of Washington Department of Urology.

Lin leads a nationwide consortium of eight institutions called the Canary Prostate Active Surveillance Study, an endeavor dedicated to identifying and validating biomarkers of high-risk prostate cancer.

Because many prostate cancers are slow growing and never become life threatening, many men with early stage prostate cancer choose active surveillance – delaying treatment while closely monitoring to see whether the cancer progresses.

Two urine-based biomarkers were found to correlate with indicators of aggressive disease: tumor volume (the number of biopsy samples that contain cancer) and Gleason score (predicting the aggressiveness of cancer by how it looks under a microscope). The markers that mirrored these correlates of disease aggressiveness were:

PCA3 – a non-coding RNA that is found at high levels in prostate cancer relative to benign prostate cells; and TMPRSS2-ERG – the fusion of TMPRSS2, a gene that is regulated by androgens, with ERG, an oncogene. These genetic rearrangements are found in about half of all prostate cancers and are thought to play a role in prostate cancer development.

The findings were based on an interim analysis of data collected from 401 men who opted for active surveillance of their cancer. The study compared biomarker performance to clinical data collected at the time of study entry. Ultimately, the study aims to enroll 1,000 men and follow them for at least five years.

"The ultimate goal is that men on active surveillance could use a test based on these biomarkers or others to complement biopsy and PSA data to indicate or rule out the presence of an undetected aggressive cancer or future development of aggressive cancer," said Lin, who cautioned that these initial results, while promising, need to be confirmed in a larger study that would evaluate changes in these urine biomarkers over time, along with correlation to disease progression during active surveillance. Lin further noted that neither PCA3 nor TMPRSS2-ERG are FDA-approved for prostate cancer detection and that their use in active surveillance is investigational.

Prostate Cancer Study Proves Drug Delays Disease Progression

For men diagnosed with low-risk, localized prostate cancer, being treated with the drug dutasteride ("Avodart") delays disease progression and initiating active treatment, and also reduces anxiety, show the results of a three-year international clinical trial led by Dr. Neil Fleshner, Head of the Division of Urology, University Health Network (UHN).

The findings are published online January 2012 in *The Lancet*. "The results prove that using active surveillance plus dutasteride is a viable, safe and effective treatment option for men who often undergo aggressive local treatment despite low risk of dying from the disease," says Dr. Fleshner, a surgical oncologist in UHN's Princess Margaret Cancer Program and Professor of Surgery at the University of Toronto. Dr. Fleshner also holds the Love Chair in Prostate Cancer Prevention Research.

"This is very good news for men with low-risk disease because aggressive treatment can have a major impact on their quality of life, with risks of impotence and incontinence," says Dr. Fleshner.

The three-year clinical trial enrolled 302 men between the ages of 48 and 82 diagnosed with low-risk localized prostate cancer and regularly monitored for clinical changes – a treatment option called "active surveillance". In the trial – known as REDEEM (REduction by

Dutasteride of clinical progression Events in Expectant Management of prostate cancer) – participants were randomized 1:1 to receive dutasteride or a matching placebo daily. The men also underwent biopsies at 1.5 and three years.

The study showed a significant delay in disease progression in the men treated with dutasteride – 38% compared with 48% who received the placebo. As well, the final biopsies showed the men treated with the drug were less likely to have cancer detected – 36% compared with 23%.

"This is the first study to show that a 5a-reductase inhibitor such as dutasteride reduces the need for aggressive treatment in low-risk disease," says Dr. Fleshner. "The drug, currently commonly used to treat enlarged prostate, works by inhibiting the male sex hormone that causes the enlargement in the first place."

Dr. Fleshner says a small percentage of men reported drug-related side effects including sexual difficulty with either desire or erections (5%), or breast tenderness or enlargement (3%). "It's important to realize that these drugs have been around for almost 20 years in clinical practice to treat enlarged prostates and so we have a wealth of knowledge about their side effects, which are reversible if the drug is stopped."

Participants were also assessed for cancer-related anxiety and the men on dutasteride reported feeling much less anxious because their biopsies and PSA values improved, adds Dr. Fleshner. (PSA – or prostate-specific antigen – is a blood test used to help diagnose prostate cancer.)

Panel endorses active monitoring and delay of treatment for low-risk prostate cancer

An independent panel convened this week by the National Institutes of Health has concluded that many men with localized, low-risk prostate cancer should be closely monitored, permitting treatment to be delayed until warranted by disease progression. However, monitoring strategies—such as active surveillance—have not been uniformly studied and available data do not yet point to clear follow-up protocols. The panel recommended standardizing definitions and conducting additional studies to clarify which monitoring strategies are most likely to optimize patient outcomes.

"It's clear that many men would benefit from delaying treatment, but there is no consensus on what constitutes observational strategies and what criteria should be used to determine when treatment might ultimately be needed among closely-monitored men," said Dr. Patricia A. Ganz, conference panel chairperson and director of the Division of Cancer Prevention and Control Research at the Jonsson Comprehensive Cancer Center at the University of California in Los Angeles.

Prostate cancer is the most common non-skin cancer in men in the United States. It is estimated that in 2011, approximately 240,000 men will be newly diagnosed with prostate cancer and 33,000 will die of the disease. More than half of these cancers are localized (confined to the prostate), not aggressive at diagnosis, and unlikely to become life-threatening. However, approximately 90 percent of patients receive immediate treatment, such as surgery or radiation therapy. For many of these patients, treatment has substantial short- and long-term side effects, such as diminished sexual function and loss of urinary control, without clear benefits, such as improved survival. Identifying appropriate management strategies for different subgroups of patients is critical to improving survival and reducing the burden of adverse effects.

Currently, clinicians often describe two alternatives to immediate treatment of low-risk prostate cancer: observation with and without the intent to cure. Observation without intent to cure, sometimes referred to as watchful waiting, is a passive approach, with treatment provided to alleviate symptoms if they develop. Observation with intent to cure, often referred to as active surveillance, involves proactive patient follow-up in which blood samples, digital rectal exams, and repeat prostate biopsies are conducted on a regular schedule, and curative treatment is initiated if the cancer progresses.

The panel identified emerging consensus in the medical community on a definition for low-risk prostate cancer: a prostate-specific antigen (PSA) level less than 10 ng/mL and a Gleason score of 6 or less. Using this definition, the panel estimated that more than 100,000 men diagnosed with prostate cancer each year would be candidates for active monitoring rather than immediate treatment. Importantly, however, the panel found that protocols to manage active monitoring still vary widely, hampering the evaluation and comparison of research findings.

Prostate cancer affects some 30-40 percent of men over the age of 50. Some of these men will benefit from immediate treatment, others will benefit from observation. We need to standardize definitions, group patients by their risks, and conduct additional research to determine the best protocols for managing low-risk disease," stated Dr. Ganz.

The panel further recommended that disease terminology should be refined as a result of changes in the patient population with prostate cancer due to prostate-specific antigen (PSA) testing. Because of the very favorable prognosis of PSA-detected, low-risk prostate cancer, the panel recommended that strong consideration be given to removing the anxiety-provoking term "cancer" for this condition.

The panel also found that clinicians' framing of disease management options is an important factor in patient decision-making. Other influential factors include views of family members, cancer experiences of family and friends, lifestyle priorities, and personal philosophy.

Findings from studies in communication sciences and behavioral economics could be applied in clinical settings to promote informed, shared decision-making. While research continues to fill knowledge gaps and develop consensus, the decisions faced by men and their providers following a diagnosis of localized, low-risk prostate cancer should be highly individualized, and include the consideration of biological, psychological, social, and cultural factors.

Chemotherapy

Prostate cancer drug delivers benefits before chemotherapy

A drug used to treat men with late-stage prostate cancer proved effective in stemming progression of the disease in research participants who had not yet received chemotherapy and extended their survival, according to results from a multi-national Phase III clinical trial led by the Knight Cancer Institute at Oregon Health & Science University (OHSU).

A comprehensive analysis of the study's results _ published in June 1 online edition of the New England Journal of Medicine and to be presented at the American Society of Clinical Oncology (ASCO) annual meeting in Chicago _ found participants treated with enzalutamide saw an 81 percent reduction in the risk the cancer would progress and a 29 percent reduction in the risk of death. The oral medication, which is marketed under the brand name Xtandi®, also helped prevent the spread of the disease to the bones, delayed the need for chemotherapy, and reduced evidence of prostate cancer in the bloodstream.

"Based on the study results, this drug could fill an important gap in prostate cancer treatment today. The strong response to this new use of enzalutamide shows that it can provide a viable, less toxic alternative to chemotherapy in staving off the disease in men who aren't responding to standard first line hormonal treatments," said Tomasz Beer, M.D., the lead author on the study and deputy director of the Knight Cancer Institute at OHSU.

The double blind Phase III study included 1,717 research participants enrolled at 207 sites globally between September 2010 and September 2012; 872 received enzalutamide while the others received a placebo. All enrolled patients had metastatic prostate cancer that was worsening despite treatment with traditional hormone therapy. None had yet received chemotherapy.

The trial, named PREVAIL, was concluded early, after a planned interim analysis, because of overwhelming response to the treatment. At this point, 72 percent of enzalutamide patients and 63 percent of placebo patients were alive at the trial cutoff date showing a 29 percent overall improvement in survival. Fatigue and hypertension were among the most common clinically relevant side effects.

Prostate cancer is the most common form of cancer in men and the second leading cause of cancer-related death in the US and the sixth leading cause of cancer-related death among men worldwide. Hormone therapies are used to treat prostate cancer patients whose disease either isn't responding to radiation or surgery or has already spread beyond the prostate gland. Male hormones, called androgens, cause prostate cancer cells to grow. Hormone therapies, known as androgen deprivation therapies, help arrest the disease by reducing a patient's androgen levels. Enzalutamide works differently than other hormone therapies; rather than reducing hormone levels, it blocks hormone binding to the androgen receptor – an essential step in hormone action

"In the past few years we have vastly expanded treatment options for prostate cancer," Beer said. "We are working hard to provide answers and options for men whose disease still resists treatment. The results of this clinical trial are extremely gratifying because they represent a leap forward for those patients."

Beer's team of prostate cancer researchers at OHSU's Knight Cancer Institute have been involved in, or led, clinical trials for three of the five new treatments developed for prostate cancer in recent years.

Enzalutamide, which is taken as four pills once per day, is already approved by the Food and Drug Administration (FDA) for men whose disease has not been stopped by other treatments including, surgery, radiation, androgen deprivation therapy and chemotherapy.

Drug combination extends survival by more than a year in metastatic prostate cancer

Men with newly diagnosed metastatic, hormone-sensitive prostate cancer lived more than a year longer when they received a chemotherapy drug as initial treatment instead of waiting to for the disease to become resistant to hormone-blockers, report scientists from Dana-Farber Cancer Institute and the Eastern Cooperative Oncology Group.

The dramatic results in a multi-center phase III trial should change the way physicians have routinely treated such patients since the 1950s, they said.

"This is the first study to identify a strategy that prolongs survival in newly diagnosed, metastatic prostate cancer," said Christopher J. Sweeney, M.B.B.S, of Dana-Farber's Lank Center for Genitourinary Oncology. He presented the results of the trial Sunday, June 1, 2014 at the annual meeting of the American Society of Clinical Oncology (ASCO) in Chicago.

"The benefit is substantial and warrants this being a new standard treatment for men who have high-extent disease and are fit for chemotherapy," added Sweeney, principal investigator of the E3805 National Cancer Institute-funded study.

"The prolongation in survival seen in the prostate cancer patients participating in Dr. Sweeney's study is very impressive, dramatically longer than the typical 2-6 month prolongation typically observed in successful studies of other metastatic adult solid tumors," said Bruce E. Johnson, MD, Dana-Farber's chief clinical research officer.

In current practice, men newly diagnosed with prostate cancer that has spread widely, and whose cancer depends on male hormones to grow, are started on hormone-blocking medications – androgen deprivation therapy (ADT). Most tumors eventually outgrow their need for hormones and the cancer progresses. Only then do patients begin chemotherapy.

The new trial tested Sweeney's hypothesis that immediately hitting the cancer with chemotherapy in addition to hormone treatment would impair the tumor cells' ability to repair damage, delaying the development of resistance.

The study enrolled 790 men newly diagnosed with metastatic disease; they were randomized to receive ADT alone or ADT with docetaxel (brand name Taxotere®) over 18 weeks. In the ADT-only group, 124 patients were given docetaxel when their cancer worsened. In the ADT-plus-docetaxel group, 45 patients whose disease progressed received additional docetaxel.

At a median follow-up of 29 months, 136 patients in the ADT-only group had died versus 101 in the group that received both drugs. This translated into a median overall survival of 57.6 months for men who received early chemotherapy compared with 44 months in the group given ADT as the only initial treatment – more than a year of additional life.

In the 520 patients who had high-extent disease (whose cancer had spread to major organs and/or the bones), treatment with ADT plus docetaxel had an even greater benefit: these men had a median overall survival of 49.2 months versus 32.2 in the ADT-only group – a difference of 17 months.

Earlier results of the trial were made public by the NCI in December 2013 because of the strong positive findings. Sweeney's presentation at ASCO covers updated and more detailed results.

Most of the striking survival benefit with early use of docetaxel was found in men with a high burden of metastatic disease. Sweeney said more time is needed to assess the benefit of the drug combination in the men with lesser burdens of disease, as their median survival has not yet been reached.

The most serious side effects were neutropenic fever and neuropathy; one patient died as a result of treatment.

The addition of docetaxel not only lengthened survival but delayed disease progression as measured by an increase in prostate-specific antigen (PSA), the appearance of new metastases, or worsening symptoms. The men receiving docetaxel had an average of 32.7 months before the cancer progressed by worsening scan results or symptoms, compared to 19.8 months for hormone therapy alone.

"This study shows that early chemotherapy increases the chances that certain patients with metastatic prostate cancer have a longer time without symptoms from cancer, and also live longer," Sweeney said.

Golden Age of Prostate Cancer Treatment Hailed as Fourth Drug in Two Years Extends Life

The head of one of the UK's leading cancer research organisations has hailed a golden age in prostate cancer drug discovery as for the fourth time in two years results are published finding a new drug can significantly extend life.

A study in the New England Journal of Medicine August 15 shows the drug enzalutamide can significantly extend life and improve quality of life in men with advanced prostate cancer -- in findings that could further widen the treatment options for men with the disease.

The Institute of Cancer Research, London, and its partner hospital The Royal Marsden NHS Foundation Trust jointly led the new Phase III trial of enzalutamide and the Phase III trials of two other drugs, cabazitaxel and abiraterone. Abiraterone was also discovered at The Institute of Cancer Research and was recently made available on the NHS. A further drug sipuleucel-T has also been shown to extend life in the two-year period.

Professor Alan Ashworth, chief executive of The Institute of Cancer Research (ICR), said cancer research in the UK was finally delivering new treatment options for men with advanced prostate cancer after a long period where the options were limited.

Professor Ashworth said: "Advanced prostate cancer is extremely difficult to treat, and it's taken a massive coordinated effort to finally bring new drugs into the pipeline, after decades where there were no options once old-style hormone treatment stopped working.

"What we're seeing now is an unprecedented period of success for prostate cancer research, with four new drugs shown to extend life in major clinical trials in just two years, and several others showing promise. It truly is a golden age for prostate cancer drug discovery and development."

Professor Martin Gore, medical director of The Royal Marsden Hospital, said: "We are delighted with the recent progress that has been made in the treatment of advanced prostate cancer and to see the impact this is having on our patients, many of whom are living longer with a better quality of life as the result of these new drugs."

Enzalutamide, a new type of hormone treatment, was assessed in 1,199 patients with metastatic castration-resistant prostate cancer that had previously received chemotherapy, in a multinational, randomised placebo-controlled trial sponsored by pharmaceutical companies Medivation and Astellas.

Median survival with enzalutamide was 18.4 months, compared with 13.6 months for men receiving a placebo. Around 43 per cent of men taking enzalutamide as part of the AFFIRM trial reported an improved quality of life, compared with 18 per cent of men taking a placebo. In November last year, the trial's Independent Data Monitoring Committee recommended that the trial be stopped early and men who received the placebo be offered enzalutamide.

Fasting may help protect against immune-related effects of chemotherapy and aging

While chemotherapy can save lives, it can also cause many side effects, including the depletion of immune cells. Also, even in the absence of chemotherapy, normal aging takes a heavy toll on the immune system, leading to immune deficiencies and a higher risk of developing leukemia and a variety of malignancies with age. Now researchers reporting in the June 5th 2014 issue of the Cell Press journal Cell Stem Cell have found that a simple dietary intervention—periodic fasting—may combat both chemotherapy-induced and aging-related changes in immune cell function by replenishing stem cells in the blood. The findings suggest that fasting may provide benefits for cancer patients, the elderly, and people with various immune defects.

It's estimated that more than one-fifth of cancer-related deaths are hastened, or even caused, by toxic effects of chemotherapy rather than the cancer itself. These toxicities can reduce the overall effectiveness of anticancer treatments by limiting the dosage and frequency of chemotherapeutic interventions that are tolerable to patients. Currently there are no interventions to lessen the side effects that chemotherapy has on the immune system or to prevent the immune cell dysfunction that occurs with aging.

Previous work by Dr. Valter Longo, of the University of Southern California, and his colleagues revealed that temporary nutrient restriction could increase stem cells' resistance to certain stressors. In their latest work, they tested whether fasting could have protective effects for immune cells such as white blood cells. "We show that prolonged fasting periods cause a major reduction in white blood cell number followed by its replenishment after refeeding," said Dr. Longo. "We discovered that this effect, which may have evolved to reduce energy expenditure during periods of starvation, is able to switch stem cells to a mode able to not only regenerate immune cells and reverse the immunosuppression caused by chemotherapy, but also rejuvenate the immune system of old mice." The researchers found that protection against white blood cell loss also occurred in human patients who fasted for a single 72-hour period prior to platinum-based chemotherapy as part of a phase 1 clinical trial.

With additional experiments, the investigators discovered that fasting provides its protective effects by reducing levels of insulin-like growth factor-1 (IGF-1), a protein with key roles in growth and aging. Therefore, fasting or treatments that target the IGF-1 pathway might provide similar benefits for cancer patients, the elderly, and people with immune defects. "We and others are currently testing the effect of fasting-mimicking diets on the protection of patients against chemotherapy's side effects, and we're also testing the role of multiple cycles of a fasting-mimicking diet on the immune system in generally healthy middle-aged and elderly subjects," said Dr. Longo.

Gene therapy

Gene therapy reduces the rate of positive prostate biopsy

Combining oncolytic adenovirus-mediated cytotoxic gene therapy (OAMCGT) with intensity modulated radiation therapy (IMRT) reduces the risk of having a positive prostate biopsy two years after treatment in intermediate-risk prostate cancer without affecting patients' quality of life, according to a study published in the June 1, 2014 edition of the *International Journal of Radiation Oncology* • Biology • Physics (Red Journal), the official scientific journal of the American Society for Radiation Oncology (ASTRO).

Previous prospective clinical trials in prostate cancer have shown that increasing the standard radiation dose of 70 Gy by 10 to 15 percent improves the biochemical disease-free survival in some prognostic risk groups; however, more than 25 percent of men with intermediate- or high-risk disease develop prostate-specific antigen (PSA) progression within 10 years, suggesting that radiation doses higher than 80 Gy may be necessary. This prospective randomized phase II trial examines the use of OAMCGT to improve the effectiveness of IMRT without increasing the radiation dose in intermediate-risk prostate cancer.

Based on encouraging results from a prior phase I trial, 44 patients were enrolled in this randomized phase II trial from January 2008 to July 2010. Patients were randomized to receive either OAMCGT with IMRT (21) or IMRT alone (23), and outcomes were focused on toxicity, quality of life and prostate biopsy findings at two years post-treatment. Eligible patients had newly diagnosed, clinically localized, intermediate-risk prostate cancer, defined as clinical stage T1/T2 with a Gleason score of 7 or a PSA of 10 to 20 ng/ml. Patients with a Gleason score of 5/6, a PSA <10 ng/ml and ≥50 percent positive biopsy cores were also eligible because it has been found that these patients tend to respond biochemically similar to patients with intermediate-risk disease. Of the 44 patients analyzed in this study, 82 percent (36) had stage T1 disease and 18 percent (8) had stage T2 disease. Sixteen percent (7) had a Gleason score of 6 and 84 percent (37) had a Gleason score of 7.

All patients were treated with IMRT (80 Gy in 2.0 Gy fractions over eight weeks). Patients who were treated with OAMCGT in addition to IMRT also received a single intraprostatic injection of 1 x 1012 viral particles of the Ad5-yCD/mutTKSR39rep-ADP adenovirus on the first day of treatment. Two days later, patients in the OAMCGT arm began IMRT treatment and received 5-FC (150 mg/kg/day, four times per day) and vGCV (1,800 mg/kg/day, twice daily) orally five days a week for two weeks.

Toxicity was assessed once a week during treatment. After completion of treatment, follow-up was conducted every three months for the first year post-treatment, at 18 and 24 months and then annually thereafter. Quality of life (QOL) was assessed at six, 12, 24 and 36 months post-treatment using the validated Expanded Prostate Cancer Index Composite (EPIC) and EuroQol EQ-5D instruments. A 12-core prostate biopsy was taken at 24 months post-treatment. Biopsies were examined by two pathologists blinded to the study treatments.

Gastrointestinal (GI) and genitourinary (GU) toxicity are the most common side effects of prostate radiation therapy. In this study, 5 percent of men (1) in the OAMCGT arm and 9 percent (2) in the IMRT alone arm experienced grade 2 or higher acute ($\leq$90 days) GI toxicity. Grade 2 or higher acute GU toxicity was more prevalent in both arms, with 43 percent (9) in the OAMCGT arm and 31 percent (7) in the IMRT alone arm; however, there was no statistical significance in acute GI or GU toxicity between the two arms. Men in the OAMCGT arm experienced a higher occurrence of influenza-like symptoms, which were expected and attributed to the oncolytic adenovirus.

The sole significant difference in QOL in the EPIC domains (urinary incontinence, unitary irritation/obstruction, bowel, sexual, hormonal and overall satisfaction) at six months post-treatment was the sexual domain, which was better in the OAMCGT arm. The only significant difference in the EQ-5D domains (mobility, self-care, usual activities, pain and discomfort, anxiety and depression, and health state) was self-care at 24 months post-treatment, which was better in the OAMCGT arm.

An important outcome was prostate biopsy at two years post-treatment, which is prognostic of long-term results. In this study, 84 percent (37) of patients had two-year biopsies. For men in the OAMCGT arm, there was a 42 percent relative reduction in positive biopsy at two years, and a 60 percent relative reduction in men with <50 percent positive biopsy cores at baseline. At the time of this study's findings, one patient in each arm had exhibited biochemical failure (4.8 percent in the OAMCGT arm and 4.3 percent in the IMRT alone arm). The events occurred 14.5 months post-treatment in the OAMCGT arm and 13.8 months post-treatment in the IMRT alone arm. No patients had developed hormone-refractory or metastatic disease, and no patients died from prostate cancer.

"The study's results demonstrate that gene therapy generated few noticeable side effects and did not diminish the patient's quality of life when combined with modern radiation therapy. Moreover, a greater percentage of men who received gene therapy and radiation had negative prostate biopsies two years after treatment relative to men who received radiation alone," said Svend O. Freytag, PhD, lead author of the study and division head of biology research in the department of radiation oncology at Henry Ford Hospital in Detroit. "Our findings suggest that gene therapy has a potential role as a strategy to enhance outcomes, along with radiation therapy, while maintaining quality of life for our patients. This research helps open the door for further studies of this novel combination therapy approach in prostate cancer and other disease sites."

Hormone Therapy

Hormone therapy may be hazardous for men with heart conditions

Adding hormone therapy to radiation therapy has been proven in randomized clinical trials to improve overall survival for men with intermediate- and high-risk prostate cancer. However, adding hormone therapy may reduce overall survival in men with pre-existing heart conditions, even if they have high-risk prostate cancer according to a new study just published online in advance of print July, 2011 in the *International Journal of Radiation Oncology•Biology•Physics*, the official scientific journal of ASTRO.

From 1991 to 2006, 14,594 men with prostate cancer were treated with brachytherapy-based radiation therapy. Of these, 1,378 (9.4 percent) had a history of congestive heart failure or myocardial infarction. Among these men with heart conditions, 22.6 percent received supplemental external beam radiation therapy and 42.9 percent received four months of androgen deprivation therapy to reduce testosterone in their bodies, which can help the cancer grow.

For the entire group of men with a history of heart problems, adding hormone therapy led to a significant increase in overall mortality. For men with pre-existing heart conditions and high-risk prostate cancer, researchers found that by 5 years, 31.8 percent of the men who received hormones had died compared to 19.5 percent of the men who did not receive hormone therapy.

"We found that for men with localized prostate cancer and a history of heart problems, treatment with hormones plus radiation was associated with a higher all-cause mortality than treatment with radiation alone, even for patients with high-risk malignant disease," Paul L. Nguyen, M.D., lead author of the study and a radiation oncologist at the Dana-Farber/Brigham and Women's Cancer Center in Boston, said. "Despite Phase III data supporting hormone therapy use for men with high-risk disease, the subgroup of men with a history of heart disease may be harmed by hormone therapy."

He added, "Future research is necessary to understand the mechanisms of this effect. In the meantime, I encourage men with prostate cancer and a history of heart disease to talk to their doctor about the benefits and risks of hormone therapy."

Some Prostate Cancer Patients Might Safely Delay Hormonal Therapy: Study

Hormone-depletion therapy is a common treatment for prostate cancer, but one that also carries side effects for men such as sexual dysfunction and fatigue. However, a new study suggests that in certain cases the treatment can be delayed -- boosting the patient's quality of life.

Doctors often track blood levels of a tumor-associated protein called prostate-specific antigen (PSA) after prostate cancer surgery or radiation therapy, to gauge whether the cancer is rebounding or not.

In the new study, researchers found that it was safe to delay hormone-depleting therapy in men with rising PSA levels who did not experience symptoms or have evidence of a tumor.

One expert applauded the study. "In view of the cost and potential side effects that are associated with hormonal therapy, this is an important study that supports the notion that we don't have to jump on early hormonal therapy if PSA is showing signs of recurrence," said Dr. Ash Tewari, chair of urology at the Icahn School of Medicine at Mount Sinai, in New York City.

The study was released at the annual meeting of the American Society of Clinical Oncology (ASCO.

"Hormone [-depleting] therapy is one of the oldest, most common and most effective treatment approaches in prostate cancer, and these findings will influence the treatment of thousands of patients worldwide," ASCO president-elect Dr. Peter Yu said in a society news release.

"This study is also a great example of how less-aggressive treatment can sometimes offer patients optimal outcomes while sparing them from side effects that impair their quality of life," Yu added.

Natural hormones such as testosterone are known to be associated with the growth of prostate tumors. So, one common treatment, called androgen deprivation therapy, involves reducing a patient's levels of these hormones.

However, ASCO experts note that the therapy also has side effects, including sexual dysfunction, weakening bones, hot flashes, fatigue, decreased mental sharpness, depression and loss of muscle mass, among others.

But what if the therapy could be at least delayed, even if a patient's PSA levels are rising? The new study found that, in certain cases, delaying hormonal therapy in this scenario is possible.

In the study, the researchers looked at data on more than 14,000 patients. Of these, just over 2,000 saw their PSA levels begin to climb again after prostate surgery or radiation therapy. These "PSA relapse" patients were divided into two groups: those who received hormone therapy immediately and those who deferred their hormone therapy until later.

The "immediate" group received hormone-depleting therapy within three months of their PSA relapse. The "deferred" group did not receive it until they developed a tumor or symptoms. Men in the "deferred" group also received hormonal therapy if their PSA level doubled in a short period of time.

Overall, the average time from initial treatment to PSA

relapse was a little more than 2 years, the researchers said. After experiencing a relapse, the men were followed for an average of almost 3.5 years.

Waiting longer to begin hormone therapy did *not* have a significant effect on men's long-term survival, the researchers reported. The estimated five-year survival for the "immediate" treatment group was about 85 percent, compared to just over 87 percent for the "deferred" group -- not a significant difference. The researchers concluded there was no significant benefit to starting hormone therapy right away after a PSA relapse.

Postponing treatment could, however, reduce the side effects and costs linked with hormone therapy. Waiting to begin treatment could give men two or more years of life without some of the common and distressing symptoms tied to the therapy, the researchers suggested.

"Rising PSA levels trigger a lot of anxiety, and many men want to start treatment as soon as possible," study lead author Dr. Xabier Garcia-Albeniz, a research associate at Harvard University School of Public Health in Boston, said in the ASCO news release.

"These findings suggest that there may be no need to rush to androgen deprivation therapy. If our results are confirmed in randomized trials, patients could feel more comfortable waiting until they develop symptoms or signs of cancer that are seen on a scan, before initiating [treatment]," Garcia-Albeniz explained.

On-and-off approach to hormone treatment may compromise survival

Taking a break from hormone-blocking prostate cancer treatments once the cancer seems to be stabilized is not equivalent to continuing therapy, a new large-scale international study finds.

Based on previous smaller studies, it looked like an approach called intermittent androgen deprivation therapy might be just as good as continuous androgen deprivation in terms of survival while meanwhile giving patients a breather from the side effects of therapy. In fact, researchers believed intermittent therapy might help overcome treatment resistance that occurs in most patients with metastatic hormone-sensitive prostate cancer.

But this new study, which treated 1,535 patients with metastatic prostate cancer and followed them for a median of 10 years, finds that's not the case. Results appear in the *New England Journal of Medicine.*

"We tried to see whether intermittent androgen deprivation is as good as continuous androgen deprivation, but we did not prove that. We found that intermittent therapy is certainly not better and moreover we cannot even call it comparable," says lead study author Maha Hussain, M.D., FACP, a prostate cancer expert oncologist at the University of Michigan Comprehensive Cancer Center.

The study was sponsored by SWOG, a National Cancer Institute-supported cancer clinical trials cooperative group.

In the study, men with metastatic hormone-sensitive prostate cancer were given an initial course of androgen deprivation therapy (hormone therapy), which is standard therapy for this disease. Patients with a stable or declining PSA level equal to or below a cut-off of 4 ng/ml were then randomly assigned either to continue or to discontinue the hormone therapy. Patients were carefully monitored with monthly PSAs and a doctor's evaluation every three months and therapy was resumed in the intermittent arm when PSA climbed to 20 ng/ml. The intermittent cycle continued on-and-off based on the PSA levels.

Survival among the two groups showed a 10 percent relative increase in the risk of death with intermittent therapy, with average survival of 5.8 years for the continuous group and 5.1 years for the intermittent group from the time of randomization.

Further, the researchers looked at quality of life between the two groups of patients. Initially the intermittent therapy group showed significant improvement in impotence and emotional function in the first three months and had improved trends in other aspects of quality of life compared to the continuous group. But these differences leveled off over time.

"The improvements in some aspects of quality of life that were observed early were not sustained after a few months as patients had to resume therapy," says Hussain professor of internal medicine and urology at the U-M Medical School.

"If a patient is coming in with newly metastatic prostate cancer, hormone treatment continuously is the standard. If they wish to do intermittent treatment, they should be counseled that based on this data, their outcome might be compromised," she adds.

Intermittent Hormone Therapy for Prostate Cancer Inferior to Continuous Therapy

Many men with metastatic, hormone-sensitive prostate cancer live longer on continuous androgen-deprivation therapy (also known as hormone therapy) than on intermittent therapy, according to a seventeen-year study led by SWOG, a cancer research cooperative group funded by the National Cancer Institute (NCI).

Men with newly diagnosed metastatic prostate cancer are usually either surgically castrated or given medications to suppress the production of male hormones that drive their cancer. The treatment can help keep the disease at bay temporarily, but in the majority of patients the cancer will relapse and contribute to the patient's death.

Surgical castration is permanent but "medical castration" provides men the potential advantage of receiving therapy intermittently. A halt in this therapy is followed in time by a rise in testosterone levels. Scientific data suggested that intermittent treatment may delay the cancer relapse, and that the rise in testosterone may result in an improvement in the patient's quality of life.

These data provided the rationale for the phase III clinical trial SWOG-9346, the largest such study to date in men with metastatic, hormone-sensitive disease. Results of this study demonstrate that intermittent androgen-deprivation (AD) therapy is not as good as continuous hormone therapy with regard to patient longevity.

"Based on these results," Hussain says, "we can conclude that intermittent AD is not as effective as continuous AD in men with metastatic prostate cancer."

Clinical researchers from the SWOG network, with funding from the NCI, led an international team in conducting the study at more than 500 sites, enrolling 3,040 men with hormone-sensitive, metastatic prostate cancer between 1995 and 2008.

All men got an initial course of androgen-deprivation treatment for seven months. The 1,535 eligible men whose prostate-specific antigen (PSA) level dropped to 4 ng/mL or less by the end of those seven months were then assigned at random to stop therapy (the intermittent therapy group) or continue therapy.

Those randomized to the intermittent therapy arm had their treatment suspended until their PSA rose to a predetermined level, at which time they started another seven-month course of androgen-deprivation therapy, cycling on and off therapy in this way as long as their PSA levels continued to respond appropriately during the "on" cycle.

Men on continuous therapy had a median overall survival time of 5.8 years from the time of randomization, with 29 percent of these men surviving at least 10 years. Those on intermittent therapy had a median overall survival time of 5.1 years, with 23 percent surviving at least 10 years from the time they were randomly assigned to a treatment arm.

The researchers found, in additional analyses, that men with "minimal disease" (disease that had not spread beyond the lymph nodes or the bones of the spine or pelvis) did significantly better on continuous therapy, while men with "extensive disease" (disease that had spread beyond the spine, pelvis, and lymph nodes or to the lungs or liver) seemed to do about as well using either treatment approach.

Additional analyses indicated that the median overall survival time for those with minimal disease was 7.1 years on continuous androgen-deprivation therapy compared to only 5.2 years on intermittent treatment.

Patients with extensive disease had median overall survival times of 4.4 years on continuous therapy and 5.0 years on intermittent therapy.

"In the past when it came to using hormone therapy in this disease, doctors viewed the disease as one entity and adopted a 'one size fits all' approach," Hussain says. "Based on this study's findings, it seems that one size does not necessarily fit all."

Trial researchers also compared quality-of-life measures across the two study arms during the first 15 months following patient randomization, including measures of sexual function (impotence and libido), physical and emotional function, and energy level. They found improved sexual function in men who received intermittent therapy as compared to those on continuous therapy.

"Though we see potential quality-of-life benefits with IAD," Hussain says, "from a medical perspective, the primary findings of the study demonstrating that IAD is inferior with regard to overall survival should be the primary consideration in counseling all patients who are interested in intermittent therapy and particularly those with minimal disease."

In brief:

1,535 men with metastatic, hormone-sensitive prostate cancer were randomized to intermittent androgen-deprivation (AD) therapy or continuous AD therapy after

seven months of androgen deprivation.
• When overall survival times were compared, intermittent AD was inferior to continuous AD.
• For the subset of patients with minimal disease, continuous AD was superior to intermittent AD.
• For patients with extensive disease, overall survival was comparable between intermittent and continuous AD.
• A number of quality-of-life measures got higher scores in the intermittent AD arm than the continuous AD arm.

Prostate cancer statistics: More than 240,000 men in the United States will be diagnosed with prostate cancer in 2012, according to the American Cancer Society, and more than 28,000 will die of the disease.

Supplemental Therapies

Aspirin

Aspirin reduces risk of prostate cancer mortality

Experimental evidence suggests that anticoagulants (ACs) may inhibit cancer growth and metastasis, but clinical data have been limited. This study investigated whether use of ACs was associated with the risk of death from prostate cancer.

This study, published online Aug. 27, 2012 in the *Journal of Clinical Oncology*., comprised 5,955 men in the Cancer of the Prostate Strategic Urologic Research Endeavor database with localized adenocarcinoma of the prostate treated with radical prostatectomy (RP) or radiotherapy (RT). Of them, 2,175 (37%) were receiving ACs (warfarin, clopidogrel, enoxaparin, and/or aspirin). The risk of prostate cancer-specific mortality (PCSM) was compared between the AC and non-AC groups.

AC therapy, particularly aspirin, was associated with a reduced risk of PCSM in men treated with RT or RP for prostate cancer. The association was most prominent in patients with high-risk disease.

Aspirin reduces the risk of cancer recurrence in prostate cancer patients

Some studies have shown that blood-thinning medications, such as aspirin, can reduce biochemical failure—cancer recurrence that is detected by a rising prostate-specific antigen (PSA) level—the risk of metastasis and even death in localized prostate cancer. These studies, although very telling, have all emphasized the need for more data. Now, with researchers at Fox Chase Cancer Center having concluded the largest study on this topic, and there is substantial data suggesting that aspirin improves outcomes in prostate cancer patients who have received radiotherapy.

A team led by Mark Buyyounouski, M.D., M.S., a radiation oncologist at Fox Chase, examined a database of over 2000 prostate cancer patients who underwent radiotherapy at Fox Chase between 1989 and 2006 and found that aspirin use lowers the risk of cancer recurrence. The scientists presented their findings on Sunday, May 1, 2011 at the 93rd Annual Meeting of the American Radium Society.

The team found that the 761 men who took aspirin at or after the time of radiotherapy were less likely to experience biochemical failure—as indicated by the levels of PSA—than were the 1380 men who didn't take the drug.

After 10-years from completion of treatment, 31% of the men who took aspirin developed recurrence compared with 39% of non-aspirin users (p=0.0005). There was also a 2% improvement in 10-year prostate cancer related survival associated with aspirin use with a trend toward statistical significance (p=0.07). "We know that prostate cancer has a long natural history and 15 years or more may be necessary to detect significant difference in survival," Dr. Buyyounouski explains. "Longer follow-up is needed, but these results warrant further study."

The readily available drug could be a promising supplement to radiotherapy in prostate cancer patients, and its beneficial effects may generalize to other types of cancer, Buyyounouski says. Still, he cautions that "it's a little premature to say that men need to start taking aspirin if they have a history of prostate cancer."

The optimal dose, timing, and duration of aspirin therapy, as well as potential side effects are not well understood, Buyyounouski explains. It's not clear how exactly the aspirin is helping and more research is needed to investigate this. "Its possible aspirin therapy is making the radiation more effective or preventing the cancer from spreading".

Coffee

Four or more cups of coffee a day may keep prostate cancer recurrence and progression away

Coffee consumption is associated with a lower risk of prostate cancer recurrence and progression, according to a new study by Fred Hutchinson Cancer Research Center scientists in *Cancer Causes & Control.*

Corresponding author Janet L. Stanford, Ph.D., co-director of the Program in Prostate Cancer Research in the Fred Hutch Public Health Sciences Division, conducted the study to determine whether the bioactive compounds in coffee and tea may prevent prostate cancer recurrence and delay progression of the disease.

Stanford and colleagues found that men who drank four or more cups of coffee per day experienced a 59 percent reduced risk of prostate cancer recurrence and/or progression as compared to those who drank only one or fewer cups per week.

They did not, however, find an association between coffee drinking and reduced mortality from prostate cancer, although the study included too few men who died of prostate cancer to address that issue separately.

First study to assess the link between tea and prostate cancer outcomes

Regarding tea consumption, the researchers did not find an associated reduction of prostate cancer recurrence and/or progression. The study also did not draw any conclusions regarding the impact of tea drinking on prostate-specific death.

"To our knowledge, our study is the first to investigate the potential association between tea consumption and prostate cancer outcomes," the authors wrote. "It is important to note, however, that few patients in our cohort were regular tea drinkers and the highest category of tea consumption was one or more cups per day. The association should be investigated in future studies that have access to larger populations with higher levels of tea consumption."

The population-based study involved 1,001 prostate cancer survivors, aged 35-74 years old at the time of diagnosis between 2002-2005, who were residents of King County, Wash. Participants answered questions regarding their diet and beverage consumption two years prior to prostate cancer diagnosis using a validated food frequency questionnaire, and were interviewed about demographic and lifestyle information, family history of cancer, medication use and prostate cancer screening history.

The researchers followed up with patients more than five years after diagnosis to ascertain whether the prostate cancer had recurred and/or progressed. Those who were still living, willing to be contacted and had been diagnosed with non-metastatic cancer were included in the follow-up effort.

Of the original 1,001 patients in the cohort, 630 answered questions regarding coffee intake, fit the follow-up criteria and were included in the final analysis. Of those, 61 percent of the men consumed at least one cup of coffee per day and 12 percent consumed the highest amount: four or more cups per day.

The study also evaluated daily coffee consumption in relation to prostate cancer-specific death in 894 patients using data from the initial food frequency questionnaire. After the median follow-up period of eight-and-a-half years, 125 of the men had died, including 38 specifically from prostate cancer. Daily coffee consumption was not associated with prostate cancer-specific mortality or other-cause mortality, but with few deaths these analyses were limited.

"Our study differs from previous ones because we used a composite definition of prostate cancer recurrence/progression," said first author Milan Geybels, a doctoral student at Maastricht University in the Netherlands who was a graduate student in Stanford's Prostate Studies group at Fred Hutch when the study was conducted. "We used detailed information on follow-up prostate-specific antigen levels, use of secondary treatment for prostate cancer and data from scans and biopsies to assess occurrence of metastases and cause-specific mortality during follow up. Using these detailed data, we could determine whether a patient had evidence of prostate cancer recurrence or progression."

The results are consistent with findings from Harvard's Health Professionals Follow-up Study, which found that men who drank six or more cups of coffee per day had a 60 percent decreased risk of metastatic/lethal prostate cancer as compared to coffee abstainers.

Further research is required to understand the mechanisms underlying the results of the study, but biological activities associated with consumption of phytochemical compounds found in coffee include anti-inflammatory and antioxidant effects and modulation of glucose metabolism. These naturally occurring compounds include:

Caffeine, which has properties that inhibit cell growth and encourage apoptosis, or programmed cell death. Previous studies have found that caffeine consumption may reduce the risk of several cancer types, including basal-cell carcinoma, glioma (a cancer of the brain and central nervous system) and ovarian cancer.

Additional studies needed to confirm whether coffee can prevent cancer recurrence

The researchers emphasize that coffee or specific coffee components cannot be recommended for secondary prevention of prostate cancer before the preventive effect has been demonstrated in a randomized clinical trial. Further, there's ongoing debate about which components in coffee are anti-carcinogenic, and additional large, prospective studies are needed to confirm whether coffee intake is beneficial for secondary prevention.

Coffee drinking may even be problematic for some men, Geybels said.

"Although coffee is a commonly consumed beverage, we have to point out that increasing one's coffee intake may be harmful for some men. For instance, men with hypertension may be vulnerable to the adverse effects of caffeine in coffee. Or, specific components in coffee may raise serum cholesterol levels, posing a possible threat to coronary health. Patients who have questions or concerns about their coffee intake should discuss them with their general practitioner," he said.

The investigators also noted limits to their study, which included a lack of data on how coffee consumption might have changed following diagnosis, whether the coffee that participants consumed was caffeinated or decaffeinated, and how the coffee was prepared (espresso, boiled or filtered), a factor that may affect the bioactive properties of the brew.

Coffee Consumption Associated with Reduced Risk of Advanced Prostate Cancer

While it is too early for physicians to start advising their male patients to take up the habit of regular coffee drinking, data presented at the American Association for Cancer Research Frontiers in Cancer Prevention Research Conference revealed a strong inverse association between coffee consumption and the risk of lethal and advanced prostate cancers.

"Coffee has effects on insulin and glucose metabolism as well as sex hormone levels, all of which play a role in prostate cancer. It was plausible that there may be an association between coffee and prostate cancer," said Kathryn M. Wilson, Ph.D., a postdoctoral fellow at the Channing Laboratory, Harvard Medical School and the Harvard School of Public Health.

In a prospective investigation, Wilson and colleagues found that men who drank the most coffee had a 60 percent lower risk of aggressive prostate cancer than men who did not drink any coffee. This is the first study of its kind to look at both overall risk of prostate cancer and risk of localized, advanced and lethal disease.

"Few studies have looked prospectively at this association, and none have looked at coffee and specific prostate cancer outcomes," said Wilson. "We specifically looked at different types of prostate cancer, such as advanced vs. localized cancers or high-grade vs. low-grade cancers."

Caffeine is actually not the key factor in this association, according to Wilson. The researchers are unsure which components of the beverage are most important, as coffee contains many biologically active compounds like antioxidants and minerals.

Using the Health Professionals' Follow-Up Study, the researchers documented the regular and decaffeinated coffee intake of nearly 50,000 men every four years from 1986 to 2006; 4,975 of these men developed prostate cancer over that time. They also examined the cross-sectional association between coffee consumption and levels of circulating hormones in blood samples collected from a subset of men in the cohort.

"Very few lifestyle factors have been consistently associated with prostate cancer risk, especially with risk of aggressive disease, so it would be very exciting if this association is confirmed in other studies," said Wilson. "Our results do suggest there is no reason to stop drinking coffee out of any concern about prostate cancer."

This association might also help understand the biology of prostate cancer and possible chemoprevention measures.

Statins

Statins may slow prostate growth

Statins drugs prescribed to treat high cholesterol may also work to slow prostate growth in men who have elevated PSA levels, according to an analysis led by researchers at Duke University Medical Center.

The finding, presented at the 2012 annual meeting of the American Urological Association, provides additional insight into the effects of cholesterol-lowering drugs such as statins on the prostate. Previous studies at Duke and elsewhere had found a link between statins and lower levels of PSA, a protein produced by the prostate that is often elevated by cancer or by non-lethal prostatic diseases.

In the current finding, prostatic growth rate diminished among men with elevated PSA levels who took statins, although that effect was relatively small and tapered off after about two years.

"Given that prostate enlargement is an important health problem in the United States and elsewhere, and will be a larger problem as the population ages, it's important to understand and treat its causes," said Roberto Muller, M.D., a urology fellow at Duke and lead author of the study.

Enlarged prostate, most commonly diagnosed as benign prostate hyperplasia, causes urinary problems that can escalate to bladder and kidney damage. Up to 90 percent of men over the age of 70 have some symptoms associated with enlarged prostate, according to the National Institutes of Health.

Muller and colleagues used data gathered for an unrelated, large trial originally testing whether a drug called dutasteride could help reduce the risk of prostate cancer. To test their hypothesis that statins may be associated with slower prostate growth, the researchers culled the data of more than 6,000 men, including 1,032 who also took statins.

Men on statins tended to be older than non-users, and thus were expected to have greater prostate sizes. But prostate sizes were actually similar between statin users and non-users at the start of the study. That finding provided the first suggestion that statins might affect prostate growth.

When changes in prostate growth were compared two years after the start of the trial, men in the study who took a statin drug had less prostate growth, regardless of whether they had been randomly assigned to take dutasteride or a dummy pill. Prostate growth was an average 5 percent less in men who took both a statin and dutasteride pill compared to men who took only dutasteride. For those taking a statin and a dummy pill, prostate growth was 3.9 percent less than for men taking only the placebo.

Those reductions, however, did not persist after two years.

"We don't yet understand the mechanisms that might be causing this," Muller said. "Some have suggested that statins may have anti-inflammatory properties, and inflammation has been linked to prostate growth, but this needs further study."

Muller said the findings in the current research also suggest that lifestyle choices such diet and exercise may not only affect cholesterol, but also prostate health.

"Prostate enlargement was once considered an inexorable consequence of aging and genetics, but there is growing awareness that prostate growth can be influenced by modifiable risk factors," Muller said. "In this context, the role of blood cholesterol levels and cholesterol-lowering drugs such as statins warrants further study."

Men who take statins are less likely to die from prostate cancer

Men with prostate cancer who take cholesterol-lowering drugs called statins are significantly less likely to die from their cancer than men who don't take such medication, according to study led by researchers at Fred

Hutchinson Cancer Research Center. The findings are published online May 2013 in *The Prostate.*

The study, led by Janet L. Stanford, Ph.D., co-director of the Prostate Cancer Research Program and a member of the Hutchinson Center's Public Health Sciences Division, followed about 1,000 Seattle-area prostate cancer patients. Approximately 30 percent of the study participants reported using statin drugs to control their cholesterol. After a mean follow-up of almost eight years, the researchers found that the risk of death from prostate cancer among statin users was 1 percent as compared to 5 percent for nonusers.

"If the results of our study are validated in other patient cohorts with extended follow-up for cause-specific death, an intervention trial of statin drugs in prostate cancer patients may be justified," Stanford said.

"While statin drugs are relatively well tolerated with a low frequency of serious side effects, they cannot be recommended for the prevention of prostate cancer-related death until a preventive effect on mortality from prostate cancer has been demonstrated in a large, randomized, placebo-controlled clinical trial," said first author Milan S. Geybels, M.Sc., formerly a researcher in Stanford's group who is now based at Maastricht University in The Netherlands.

The study is unique in that most prior research of the impact of statin use on prostate cancer outcomes has focused on biochemical recurrence – a rising PSA level –

and not prostate cancer-specific mortality. "Very few studies of statin use in relation to death from prostate cancer have been conducted, possibly because such analyses require much longer follow-up for the assessment of this prostate cancer outcome," Geybels said.

The potential biological explanation behind the association between statin use and decreased mortality from prostate cancer may be related to cholesterol- and non-cholesterol-mediated mechanisms.

• An example of the former: When cholesterol is incorporated into cell membranes, these "cholesterol-rich domains" play a key role in controlling pathways associated with survival of prostate cancer cells.
• An example of the latter: Statin drugs inhibit an essential precursor to cholesterol production called mevalonate. Lower levels of mevalonate may reduce the risk of fatal prostate cancer.

"Prostate cancer is an interesting disease for which secondary prevention, or preventing poor long-term patient outcomes, should be considered because it is the most common cancer among men in developed countries and the second leading cause of cancer-related deaths," Geybels said. "While many prostate cancer patients have indolent, slow-growing tumors, others have aggressive tumors that may recur or progress to a life-threatening disease despite initial therapy with radiation or surgery.

Statins associated with lower cancer recurrence following prostatectomy

Men who use statins to lower their cholesterol are 30 percent less likely to see their prostate cancer come back after surgery compared to men who do not use the drugs, according to researchers at Duke University Medical Center. Researchers also found that higher doses of the drugs were associated with lower risk of recurrence.

The findings are published in the journal *CANCER* June 2010.

"The findings add another layer of evidence suggesting that statins may have an important role in slowing the growth and progression of prostate cancer," says Stephen Freedland, M.D., a member of the Duke Prostate Center and the Urology Section at the Durham Veterans Affairs Medical Center, and the senior author of the study. "Previous studies have shown that statins have anti-cancer properties, but it's not entirely clear when it's best to use them – or even how they work."

Researchers examined the records of 1319 men who underwent radical prostatectomy included in the Shared Equal Access Regional Cancer Hospital (SEARCH) database. They found that 18 percent of the men – 236 – were taking statins at the time of surgery.

Researchers followed the patients after surgery to evaluate recurrence rates, measured by slight rises in the PSA levels after surgery, a development known as "biochemcical recurrence." Time to biochemical recurrence is viewed as an important clinical factor because it is correlated with the risk of disease progression and death.

The authors found that 304 men had a rising PSA, including 37 (16 percent) of the statin users and 267 (25 percent) of the non-users. Taking into account various clinical and pathological features that differed between the two groups, the data showed that overall, statin use reduced the risk of biochemical recurrence by 30 percent.

Among men taking statins equivalent to 20 mg of simvastatin a day, the risk of recurrence was reduced 43 percent and among the men taking the equivalent of more than 20 mg of simvastatin a day, the risk of recurrence was reduced 50 percent. Men who took a statin dose the equivalent of less than 20 mg of simvastatin daily saw no benefit.

There were significant differences between those who took the drugs and those who did not. Statin users tended to be white, older and heavier than non-users. They also had lower clinical stages at diagnosis, but higher Gleason scores, a measure of tumor aggressiveness.

"These findings are intriguing, but we do need to approach them with some caution," says Robert Hamilton, M.D., a urologist at the University of Toronto and the lead author of the study. "For example, we don't know the diet, exercise or smoking habits of these men.

So it's not entirely clear if the lower risk we detected is related to the statins alone – it could be due to other factors we were not able to measure. We do feel, however, that based on these findings and those from other studies, the time is ripe to perform a well-controlled randomized trial to test whether statins do indeed slow prostate cancer progression."

Diet and Exercise

Tomato-broccoli combo shown to be effective against prostate cancer

A new University of Illinois study shows that tomatoes and broccoli--two vegetables known for their cancer-fighting qualities--are better at shrinking prostate tumors when both are part of the daily diet than when they're eaten alone.

"When tomatoes and broccoli are eaten together, we see an additive effect. We think it's because different bioactive compounds in each food work on different anti-cancer pathways," said University of Illinois food science and human nutrition professor John Erdman.

In a study published in the January 15, 2007 issue of *Cancer Research,* Erdman and doctoral candidate Kirstie Canene-Adams fed a diet containing 10 percent tomato powder and 10 percent broccoli powder to laboratory rats that had been implanted with prostate cancer cells. The powders were made from whole foods so the effects of eating the entire vegetable could be compared with consuming individual parts of them as a nutritional supplement.

Other rats in the study received either tomato or broccoli powder alone; or a supplemental dose of lycopene, the red pigment in tomatoes thought to be the effective cancer-preventive agent in tomatoes; or finasteride, a drug prescribed for men with enlarged prostates. Another group of rats was castrated.

After 22 weeks, the tumors were weighed. The tomato/broccoli combo outperformed all other diets in shrinking prostate tumors. Biopsies of tumors were evaluated at The Ohio State University, confirming that tumor cells in the tomato/broccoli-fed rats were not proliferating as rapidly. The only treatment that approached the tomato/broccoli diet's level of effectiveness was castration, said Erdman.

"As nutritionists, it was very exciting to compare this drastic surgery to diet and see that tumor reduction was similar. Older men with slow-growing prostate cancer who have chosen watchful waiting over chemotherapy and radiation should seriously consider altering their diets to include more tomatoes and broccoli," said Canene-Adams.

How much tomato and broccoli should a 55-year-old man concerned about prostate health eat in order to receive these benefits? The scientists did some conversions.

"To get these effects, men should consume daily 1.4 cups of raw broccoli and 2.5 cups of fresh tomato, or 1 cup of tomato sauce, or _ cup of tomato paste. I think it's very doable for a man to eat a cup and a half of broccoli per day or put broccoli on a pizza with _ cup of tomato paste," said Canene-Adams.

Erdman said the study showed that eating whole foods is better than consuming their components. "It's better to eat tomatoes than to take a lycopene supplement," he said. "And cooked tomatoes may be better than raw tomatoes. Chopping and heating make the cancer-fighting constituents of tomatoes and broccoli more bioavailable."

"When tomatoes are cooked, for example, the water is removed and the healthful parts become more concentrated. That doesn't mean you should stay away from fresh produce. The lesson here, I think, is to eat a variety of fruits and vegetables prepared in a variety of ways," Canene-Adams added.

Another recent Erdman study shows that rats fed the tomato carotenoids phytofluene, lycopene, or a diet containing 10 percent tomato powder for four days had significantly reduced testosterone levels. "Most prostate cancer is hormone-sensitive, and reducing testosterone levels may be another way that eating tomatoes reduces prostate cancer growth," Erdman said.

Erdman said the tomato/broccoli study was a natural to be carried out at Illinois because of the pioneering work his colleague Elizabeth Jeffery has done on the cancer-fighting agents found in broccoli and other cruciferous vegetables. Jeffery has discovered sulfur compounds in broccoli that enhance certain enzymes in the human body, which then act to degrade carcinogens.

"For ten years, I've been learning how the phytochemicals in tomatoes affect the progression of prostate cancer. Meanwhile Dr. Jeffery has been investigating the ways in which the healthful effects of broccoli are produced. Teaming up to see how these vegetables worked together just made sense and certainly contributes to our knowledge about dietary treatments for prostate cancer," said Erdman.

Low-fat fish oil diet protects men with prostate cancer

Men with prostate cancer who ate a low-fat diet and took fish oil supplements had lower levels of pro-inflammatory substances in their blood and a lower cell cycle progression score, a measure used to predict cancer recurrence, than men who ate a typical Western diet, UCLA researchers found.

The findings are important because lowering the cell cycle progression (CCP) score may help prevent prostate cancers from becoming more aggressive, said study lead author William Aronson, a clinical professor of urology at UCLA and chief of urologic oncology at the West Los Angeles Veterans Affairs Medical Center.

"We found that CCP scores were significantly lower in the prostate cancer in men who consumed the low-fat fish oil diet as compare to men who followed a higher fat Western diet," Aronson said. "We also found that men on the low-fat fish oil diet had reduced blood levels of pro-inflammatory substances that have been associated with cancer."

This study appears in *Cancer Prevention Research,* a peer-reviewed journal of the American Association for Cancer Research.

This study is a follow-up to a 2011 study by Aronson and his team that found a low-fat diet with fish oil supplements eaten for four to six weeks prior to prostate removal slowed the growth of cancer cells in human prostate cancer tissue compared to a traditional, high-fat Western diet.

That short-term study also found that the men on the low-fat fish oil diet were able to change the composition of their cell membranes in both the healthy cells and the cancer cells in the prostate. They had increased levels of omega-3 fatty acids from fish oil and decreased levels of the more pro-inflammatory omega-6 fatty acids from corn oil in the cell membranes, which may directly affect the biology of the cells, Aronson said.

"These studies are showing that, in men with prostate cancer, you really are what you eat," Aronson said. "The studies suggest that by altering the diet, we may favorably affect the biology of prostate cancer."

The men in the previous study were placed into one of two groups, the low-fat fish oil diet or the Western diet. The Western diet consisted of 40 percent of calories from fat, generally equivalent to what many Americans consume today. The fat sources also were typical of the American diet and included high levels of omega-6 fatty acids from corn oil and low levels of fish oil that provide omega-3 fatty acids.

The low-fat diet consisted of 15 percent of calories from fat. Additionally, the men on this diet took five grams of fish oil per day in five capsules, three with breakfast and two with dinner, to provide omega-3 fatty acids. Omega-3 fatty acids have been found to reduce inflammation, and may be protective for other malignancies.

For this study, Aronson wanted to look at the potential biological mechanisms at work in the low-fat fish oil diet that may be providing protection against cancer growth and spread. They measured levels of the pro-inflammatory substances in the blood and examined the prostate cancer tissue to determine the CCP score.

"This is of great interest, as the CCP score in prostate cancer is known to be associated with more aggressive disease and can help predict which patients will recur and potentially die from their cancer," Aronson said.

Further, Aronson and his team analyzed one pro-inflammatory substance called leukotriene B4 (LTB4) and found that men with lower blood levels of LTB4 after the diet also had lower CCP scores.

"Given this finding, we went on to explore how the LTB4 might potentially affect prostate cancer cells and discovered a completely novel finding that one of the receptors for LTB4 is found on the surface of prostate cancer cells," Aronson said.

Further studies are planned to determine the importance of this novel receptor in prostate cancer progression, Aronson said.

Based on the results of his research, Aronson has been funded to start a prospective, randomized trial at UCLA next year studying 100 men who have elected to join the active surveillance program, which monitors slow-growing prostate cancer using imaging and biopsy instead of treating the disease. Study volunteers will receive a prostate biopsy at the beginning of the trial and again at one year. The men will be randomized into a group that eats their usual diet or to a low-fat fish oil diet group. Aronson will measure markers in the prostate biopsy tissue to check for cell growth and CCP score.

Prostate cancer is a leading cause of death among men in the United States. It's estimated that more than 230,000 American men will be diagnosed with prostate cancer this year alone, with more than 29,000 dying from their disease.

Oregano Kills Prostate Cancer Cells

Oregano, the common pizza and pasta seasoning herb, has long been known to possess a variety of beneficial health effects, but a new study by researchers at Long

Island University (LIU) indicates that an ingredient of this spice could potentially be used to treat prostate cancer, the second leading cause of cancer death in American men.

Prostate cancer is a type of cancer that starts in the prostate gland and usually occurs in older men. Recent data shows that about 1 in 36 men will die of prostate cancer. Estimated new cases and deaths from this disease condition in the US in 2012 alone are 241,740 and 28,170, respectively. Current treatment options for patients include surgery, radiation therapy, hormone therapy, chemotherapy, and immune therapy. Unfortunately, these are associated with considerable complications and/or severe side effects.

Dr. Supriya Bavadekar, PhD, RPh, Assistant Professor of Pharmacology at LIU's Arnold & Marie Schwartz College of Pharmacy and Health Sciences, is currently testing carvacrol, a constituent of oregano, on prostate cancer cells. The results of her study demonstrate that the compound induces apoptosis in these cells. Apoptosis, Dr. Bavadekar explains, is programmed cell death, or simply "cell suicide." Dr. Bavadekar and her group are presently trying to determine the signaling pathways that the compound employs to bring about cancer cell suicide.

"We know that oregano possesses anti-bacterial as well as anti-inflammatory properties, but its effects on cancer cells really elevate the spice to the level of a super-spice like turmeric," said Dr. Bavadekar. Though the study is at its preliminary stage, she believes that the initial data indicates a huge potential in terms of carvacrol's use as an anti-cancer agent. "A significant advantage is that oregano is commonly used in food and has a 'Generally Recognized As Safe' status in the US. We expect this to translate into a decreased risk of severe toxic effects."

"Some researchers have previously shown that eating pizza may cut down cancer risk. This effect has been mostly attributed to lycopene, a substance found in tomato sauce, but we now feel that even the oregano seasoning may play a role," stated Dr. Bavadekar. "If the study continues to yield positive results, this super-spice may represent a very promising therapy for patients with prostate cancer."

Exercise = improved prostate cancer outcomes

Men who walked at a fast pace prior to a prostate cancer diagnosis had more regularly shaped blood vessels in their prostate tumors compared with men who walked slowly, providing a potential explanation for why exercise is linked to improved outcomes for men with prostate cancer, according to results presented here at the AACR-Prostate Cancer Foundation Conference on Advances in Prostate Cancer Research.

Men who engage in higher levels of physical activity have been reported to have a lower risk of prostate cancer recurrence and mortality compared with men who participate in little or no physical activity. The biological mechanisms underlying this association are not known.

"Prior research has shown that men with prostate tumors containing more regularly shaped blood vessels have a more favorable prognosis compared with men with prostate tumors containing mostly irregularly shaped blood vessels," said Erin Van Blarigan, Sc.D., assistant professor in the Department of Epidemiology and Biostatistics at the University of California, San Francisco. "In this study, we found that men who reported walking at a brisk pace had more regularly shaped blood vessels in their prostate tumors compared with men who reported walking at a less brisk pace.

"Our findings suggest a possible mechanism by which exercise may improve outcomes in men with prostate cancer," continued Van Blarigan. "Although data from randomized, controlled trials are needed before we can conclude that exercise causes a change in vessel regularity or clinical outcomes in men with prostate cancer, our study supports the growing evidence of the benefits of exercise, such as brisk walking, for men with prostate cancer."

The Health Professionals Follow-up Study, which was initiated in 1986, enables researchers to examine how nutritional and lifestyle factors affect the incidence of serious illnesses, such as cancer and heart disease. Every two years, participants receive questionnaires that ask about diseases and health-related topics like smoking, physical activity, and medications taken. Questionnaires that ask detailed dietary information are administered every four years.

Van Blarigan and colleagues investigated whether prediagnostic physical activity was associated with prostate tumor blood vessel regularity among 572 men enrolled in the Health Professionals Follow-up Study. Prediagnostic physical activity was determined through analysis of questionnaire answers. Blood vessel regularity was established by semiautomated image analysis of the tumor samples. Blood vessels that are perfect circles are considered the ideal shape and given a score of 1. Higher values indicate less regular blood vessels.

The researchers found that men with the fastest walking pace (3.3-.5 miles per hour) prior to diagnosis had 8 percent more regularly shaped blood vessels compared with men with the slowest walking pace (1.5-.5 miles per hour).

"Our study, which provides a potential explanation by which exercise may improve outcomes in men with prostate cancer, highlights the value of multidisciplinary collaborations between laboratory, clinical, and population scientists to explore new pathways by which lifestyle factors or other exposures may affect disease," said Van Blarigan. "It is reasonable to hypothesize that the same explanation could exist for the beneficial effects of exercise in other cancers, and it would be interesting to examine this in future studies."

Football improves strength in men with prostate cancer

Research

Men with prostate cancer aged 43_74 achieve bigger and stronger muscles, improve functional capacity, gain positive social experiences and the desire to remain active through playing football for 12 weeks. These are the findings of the "FC Prostate" trial, jointly conducted by the University Hospitals Centre for Health Care Research at The Copenhagen University Hospital, Rigshospitalet and the Copenhagen Centre for Team Sport and Health at the University of Copenhagen.

Regained body pride and strong social cohesion

The acclaimed Scandinavian Journal of Medicine & Science in Sports is today publishing two articles on recreational football (soccer) for 43_74-year-old men with prostate cancer. The first article shows that twice-weekly 1-hour football training sessions for 12 weeks produce an increase in muscle mass and muscle strength despite concurrent androgen deprivation therapy. The second article describes how recreational football is a promising novel approach for health promotion in prostate cancer patients as the participants regain pride in their bodies, develop team spirit and mutual concern increasing their motivation for long-term participation in sport.

"This is the first study of its kind in the world, and the results clearly show the potential of recreational football in the rehabilitation of prostate cancer patients," says project leader Julie Midtgaard, a psychologist at The Copenhagen University Hospital Rigshospitalet. "Just 12 weeks of football training resulted in the men regaining control and developing a unique exchange of feelings and recognition centered around the sport."

The attendance rate was high over the 12 weeks, and many of the participants are still playing football two years after the project began.

"The provision of football proved to be a good way of developing friendships between the men and a unique model for men with prostate cancer to take responsibility of their own health without giving up their claim to feel and behave like men," concludes Midtgaard.

Bigger and stronger muscles in spite of anti-hormone treatment

"Androgen deprivation therapy through medical castration is an effective treatment of prostate cancer patients but has adverse effects in the form of reduced muscle mass, higher fat percentage and reduced physical activity," explains Professor Peter Krustrup, who co-initiated the study with Midtgaard and has been studying the effects of recreational football for the past 10 years.

"Twelve weeks of football training increased muscle mass by half a kilo in the football group in spite of the anti-hormone treatment and contributed to a 15% increase in muscle strength. The players in the FC Prostate team thus achieved excellent gains in functional capacity as a result of 12 weeks of football training, measured among other things as a 8% improvement in performance in the stand-sit test," says Krustrup.

"Our study also showed that recreational football was fun and inclusive for the participants in FC Prostate, and for every training session the intensity was high, with an average heart rate of 85% of the participants' maximum heart rate," says Krustrup.

Football is good rehabilitation for prostate cancer patients

"Previously, we showed that recreational football is effective for preventing and treating lifestyle diseases. With this study, we can add that recreational football can also be used for rehabilitation of a large group of cancer patients," says Krustrup.

Midtgaard concludes: "The study indicates that men with prostate cancer benefit greatly from recreational football, both physically and mentally. It has also proved to be easy to keep the men involved in physical activity once they have started playing football. They look forward to going to training and enjoy it tremendously when they get there. The next step is to evaluate the effectiveness of football in a more natural setting. Therefore we are delighted that we have received the necessary funding to pursue an even bigger project in collaboration with the Danish Football Association in which more than 300 prostate cancer patients will be invited to play football in local football clubs in Denmark."

About the study

The training project was a randomised controlled trial involving 57 men aged 67 (range: 43_74) years who had been undergoing treatment for prostate cancer for an average of 3 years. They were randomly assigned to a football training group or an inactive control group. The football group trained twice a week for 1 hour for 12 weeks.

The training took place on the football pitch of the Department of Nutrition, Exercise and Sports at Nørrebro in Copenhagen. An extensive testing protocol was used before the start of training and on completion of the 12-week training period. The project was implemented jointly by Rigshospitalet, the Copenhagen Centre for Team Sport and Health at the University of Copenhagen and the Department of Cardiology at Gentofte Hospital.

Radiation

Brachytherapy May Be An Effective Option For High-Risk Prostate Cancers

Brachytherapy for high-risk prostate cancers patients has historically been considered a less effective modality, but a new study from radiation oncologists at the Kimmel Cancer Center at Jefferson suggests otherwise. A population-based analysis looking at almost 13,000 cases revealed that men who received brachytherapy alone or in combination with external beam radiation therapy (EBRT) had significantly reduced mortality rates.

Their findings are reported online in the *International Journal of Radiation Oncology,Biology,Physics.*

Brachytherapy involves the precise placement of radiation sources directly at the site of a tumor and is typically used to treat low and intermediate risk prostate cancers. However, brachytherapy treatment for high-risk patients is less common and controversial, given in part to early retrospective studies that found it to be associated with lower cure rates compared to EBRT.

Many experts believe that these early series were limited by poor brachytherapy technique, and that high-quality contemporary brachytherapy may be an effective tool against high-risk prostate cancer.

"The study contradicts traditional policies of using brachytherapy in just low and intermediate risk patients by suggesting there may instead be an improvement in prostate cancer survival for high-risk patients," said co-author Timothy Showalter, M.D., assistant professor in the Department of Radiation Oncology at Thomas Jefferson University Hospital, and associate research member of Jefferson's Kimmel Cancer Center. "Although studies like this cannot prove an advantage for brachytherapy, our report does suggest that brachytherapy is no less effective than EBRT and should be considered for some men with high-risk prostate cancer."

Researchers identified 12,745 Surveillance, Epidemiology and End Results database patients diagnosed from 1988 to 2002 with high-grade prostate cancer of poorly differentiated grade and treated with brachytherapy (7.1 percent), EBRT alone (73.5 percent) or brachytherapy plus EBRT (19.1 percent). The team used multivariate models to examine patient and tumor characteristics associated with the likelihood of treatment with each radiation modality and the effect of radiation modality on prostate cancer-specific mortality.

Treatment with brachytherapy alone or brachytherapy in combination with EBRT, the researchers found, was associated with significant reduction in prostate cancer-specific mortality rates compared to EBRT alone.

Significant predictors of use of brachytherapy or brachytherapy plus EBRT were younger age, later year of diagnosis, urban residence and earlier T-stage.

According to the researchers, including lead author Xinglei Shen, M.D., a resident in Jefferson's Department of Radiation Oncology and a part-time master's degree student in the Jefferson School of Population Health, the study's findings provide ample evidence to further study brachytherapy as part of an effective treatment strategy for men with high-grade prostate cancer.

"Today, for the most part, brachytherapy is not being used for these high-risk patients or even recommended," Dr. Shen said. "But if you look at the biology and theory behind it, it makes sense: you can really give a lot more dose with brachytherapy than with EBRT alone to the prostate. And this presents an opportunity for high-risk patients."

Shorter radiation course for prostate cancer is effective in long-term follow-up

A shorter course of radiation treatment that delivers higher doses of radiation per day in fewer days (hypofractionation) is as effective in decreasing intermediate to high-risk prostate cancer from returning as conventional radiation therapy at five years after treatment, according to a randomized trial presented at the plenary session, October 3, 2011, at the 53rdAnnual Meeting of the American Society for Radiation Oncology (ASTRO).

"This long-term study confirms that hypofractionated radiation that shortens treatment by about two and a half weeks is a practical approach to effectively controlling prostate cancer, as compared to the more standard treatment for men with intermediate to high-risk prostate cancer," Alan Pollack, MD, chairman of radiation oncology at the University of Miami Miller School of Medicine in Miami, said.

The strategy to compress treatment schedules using hypofractionation is based on years of studies indicating that there could be a radiobiologic advantage to this approach. Prior research has indicated that tumor cells would be killed to a greater degree with hypofractionation than the potentially damaging effects on the surrounding normal tissues, namely the rectum, penile structures affecting erections and bladder. Another newer approach to hypofractionation incorporated into this trial is the use of intensity modulated radiotherapy (IMRT), which further limits dose to the normal tissues. IMRT has proven value in limiting side effects in the treatment of prostate cancer with external beam radiotherapy.

The study involved 303 men with intermediate to high-risk prostate cancer who were randomized to receive either hypofractionated IMRT or conventionally fractionated IMRT between 2002 and 2006. The high risk patients also received a form of hormone therapy for two years. The patients were followed for over five years to find out if their cancer returned by monitoring prostate specific antigen (PSA), a blood test and established indicator of prostate cancer recurrence when increasing levels are seen.

Dr. Pollack said, "we are still learning how best to apply hypofractionation and the results in this trial show that the technique is very effective."

The hypofractionation approach used was given in a shorter period of time with higher doses per day and was expected to be equivalent to four extra treatments using conventional fractionation. While the hypofractionation treatment was hypothesized to be superior, the same tumor control rates were observed. The conventionally fractionated patients had better outcomes than expected. The benefit of the hypofractionation method used was that comparable results were achieved in two and a half fewer weeks of treatment.

In terms of side effects, the rates were relatively low for both methods. There were identical long-term rates of bowel/rectal reactions and the frequency of unsatisfactory erections. There was, however, significantly higher bladder control in the conventionally fractionated patients.

"Late urinary symptoms were higher with hypofractionation but were low overall, particularly when the incidence of persistent urinary symptoms (<10 percent at five years) was analyzed, rather than just as an isolated event," Dr. Pollack said. "Hypofractionation is rapidly gaining momentum for many types of cancers.

The results presented here bring us much closer to effectively treating prostate cancer in a shorter period of time, with acceptable side effects."

Proton therapy effective prostate cancer treatment

Proton therapy, a type of external beam radiation therapy, is a safe and effective treatment for prostate cancer, according to two new studies published in the January, 2012 issue of the *International Journal of Radiation Oncology•Biology•Physics (Red Journal),* the American Society for Radiation Oncology's (ASTRO) official scientific journal.

In the first study, researchers at the University of Florida in Jacksonville, Fla., prospectively studied 211 men with low-, intermediate-, and high-risk prostate cancer. The men were treated with proton therapy, a specialized type of external beam radiation therapy that uses protons instead of X-rays. After a two year follow-up, the research team led by Nancy Mendenhall, MD, of the University of Florida Proton Therapy Institute, reported that the treatment was effective and that the gastrointestinal and genitourinary side effects were generally minimal.

"This study is important because it will help set normal tissue guidelines in future trials," Dr. Mendenhall, said.

In the second study, researchers from Massachusetts General Hospital in Boston, Loma Linda University Medical Center in Loma Linda, Calif., and the Radiation Therapy Oncology Group in Philadelphia performed a case-matched analysis comparing high-dose external beam radiation therapy using a combination of photons (X-rays) and protons with brachytherapy (radioactive seed implants).

Over three years, 196 patients received the external beam treatments. Their data was compared to 203 men of similar stages who received brachytherapy over the same time period. Researchers then compared the biochemical failure rates (a statistical measure of whether the cancer relapses) and determined that men who received the proton/photon therapy had the same rate of recurrence as the men who received brachytherapy.

"For men with prostate cancer, brachytherapy and external beam radiation therapy using photons and protons are both highly effective treatments with similar relapse rates," John J. Coen, MD, a radiation oncologist at Massachusetts General Hospital in Boston, said. "Based on this data, it is our belief that men with prostate cancer can reasonably choose either treatment for localized prostate cancer based on their own concerns about quality of life without fearing they are compromising their chance for a cure."

New radiation therapy extends life for prostate cancer patients

Prostate cancer patients with advanced tumors that have spread to bone have a poor chance of surviving. Patients with the disease may now live longer with a new line of radioisotope therapy, say researchers at the Society of Nuclear Medicine's 2012 Annual Meeting.

The skeletal system is the number one metastatic site in patients with prostate cancer. Bone metastases occur when the primary cancer is transmitted through the blood and develops in the bone. This is a phase III study for the radioisotope therapy Radium-223 chloride, or Ra-223, which seeks out bone metastases with very potent alpha particles that are deadly to tumors. The powerful drug has a short range of penetration of alpha particles, sparing nearby healthy tissues and essential bone marrow. It is initially being studied for the treatment of castration-resistant prostate cancer, a late-stage form of cancer that is typically characterized by extensive skeletal metastases that are resistant to treatment.

"This is a pivotal study of a new treatment that potentially offers a better standard of care for patients with advanced prostate cancer," says Val Lewington, professor of clinical therapeutic nuclear medicine at King's College and Guy's and St Thomas' Hospital in London, United Kingdom. "Radium-223 offers a completely new approach to the treatment of bone metastases. It systemically treats multiple sites of disease simultaneously and is usually very well tolerated.

Serious side effects are unusual, and the risk of bone marrow suppression is low even in patients who have been heavily pretreated with chemotherapy."

According to the U.S. National Cancer Institute, 241,740 new cases of prostate cancer are expected to be diagnosed and 28,170 to die from the disease this year in the United States. In the past 25 years, many bone targeted drugs have been developed to treat the disease, but they have more of a palliative effect, treating pain, but not necessarily prolonging the lives of patients.

Men with castration-resistant prostate cancer generally live three to five years after diagnosis. This double-blind and randomized study was able to show that of the 921 patients treated with either Ra-223 or a placebo, patients who received the drug lived an average of three months longer. Therapy was administered in six injections at four-week intervals. In addition to prolonged survival, those treated with Ra-223 also experienced delayed onset of complications due to bone metastases. Therapy monitoring is made possible with molecular imaging techniques called scintigraphy and positron emission tomography, which provide information about biological processes, including those involved in cancerous tumors.

An expanded access program is already underway in the United States and a similar program is expected to open in Europe in 2012. Further clinical trials are also being considered. Formal regulatory approval will be sought in mid-2012 in both the United States and Europe.

Intensity Modulated Radiation Therapy optimal for localized prostate cancer

A treatment for localized prostate cancer known as Intensity Modulated Radiation Therapy (IMRT) is better than conventional conformal radiation therapy (CRT) for reducing certain side effects and preventing cancer recurrence, according to a study published in the April 18, 2012 issue of the Journal of the American Medical Association. In 2012, approximately 241,740 American men will be diagnosed with prostate cancer.

The study also showed IMRT to be as effective as proton therapy, a newer technique that has grown in popularity in recent years.

Ronald Chen, MD, MPH, senior author, says, "Patients and doctors are often drawn to new treatments, but there have not been many studies that directly compare new radiation therapy options to older ones."

Chen is assistant professor of radiation oncology and a research fellow at the Sheps Center for Health Services Research at the University of North Carolina at Chapel Hill. He is a member of UNC Lineberger Comprehensive Cancer Center.

He explains, "In the past 10 years, IMRT has largely replaced conventional CRT as the main radiation technique for prostate cancer, without much data to support it. This study validated our change in practice, showing that IMRT better controls prostate cancer and results in fewer side effects.

"Our data show that in comparing IMRT to proton therapy, IMRT patients had a lower rate of gastrointestinal side effects, but there were no significant differences in rates of other side effects or additional therapies."

Study scientists report that compared to CRT, IMRT was associated with fewer diagnoses of gastrointestinal (GI) symptoms, such as rectal bleeding or diarrhea, hip fractures and additional cancer therapy, but more difficulty with sexual function. Proton therapy was associated with more GI problems than IMRT.

The UNC team used Surveillance, Epidemiology, and End Results (SEER)-Medicare linked data from 2000-2009 for approximately 13,000 patients with non-metastatic prostate cancer. SEER is composed of 16 population-based cancer registries representing approximately 26 percent of the US population.

This study is an example of comparative effectiveness research, which seeks to inform health care decisions by providing new research-based evidence about the benefits and harms of different health care interventions.

Tim Carey, MD, director of the Sheps Center at UNC, said, "This type of research is critical, comparing one type of treatment with alternatives, so that patients and their providers can arrive at the best decisions for each individual."

CRT, IMRT and Proton therapy represent three types of radiation, each attempting to deliver radiation treatment to a tumor while minimizing radiation dose to surrounding organs. Use of proton therapy use in prostate cancer is controversial because of its high cost and unproven benefit compared to other standard forms of radiation like IMRT.

Adverse effects among different radiation therapies for prostate cancer

In an analysis of three different types of radiation therapy used to treat localized prostate cancer, compared with conformal radiation therapy, intensity-modulated radiation therapy (IMRT) was associated with fewer diagnoses of gastrointestinal adverse effects, hip fractures, and receipt of additional cancer treatments but more erectile dysfunction, while proton therapy was associated with more gastrointestinal adverse effects than IMRT, according to a study in *JAMA*. Ronald C. Chen, M.D., M.P.H., of the University of North Carolina at Chapel Hill, presented the findings of the study.

"Prostate cancer is the most common malignancy in men, with more than 200,000 diagnoses and 30,000 deaths per year. Recent advances in technology have led to costlier treatments such as minimally invasive radical prostatectomy, intensity-modulated radiation therapy, and proton therapy. The adoption of these technologies resulted in a $350 million increase in health care expenditures in 2005 alone," according to background information in the article. Various organizations have called for comparative effectiveness research of localized prostate cancer treatments. "The clinical benefit from these newer treatments is unproven, and comparative effectiveness research examining different radiation techniques is lacking," the authors write.

Dr. Chen and colleagues conducted a study to examine the comparative adverse effects and disease control outcomes after different radiation techniques in a recent cohort of prostate cancer patients. Specifically, the researchers compared IMRT, which has been rapidly adopted and is currently the most commonly used technique, with the older conformal radiation therapy; and compared proton therapy, the use of which also has increased, with IMRT. The population-based study used Surveillance, Epidemiology, and End Results-Medicare-linked data from 2000 through 2009 for patients with localized prostate cancer. The primary outcomes measured were rates of gastrointestinal adverse effects (such as rectal bleeding or diarrhea) and urinary adverse effects, erectile dysfunction, hip fractures, and receipt of additional cancer therapy – as an indicator for disease recurrence.

The use of IMRT vs. conformal radiation therapy increased from 0.15 percent in 2000 to 95.9 percent in 2008. In the propensity-score adjusted analysis (n =

12,976), the researchers found that men treated with IMRT were less likely to receive a diagnosis of gastrointestinal adverse effects and hip fracture but more likely to receive a diagnosis of erectile dysfunction. Also, IMRT patients were nearly 20 percent less likely to receive additional cancer therapy.

In a propensity score-matched comparison between IMRT and proton therapy (n = 1,368), IMRT patients had a 34 percent lower risk of gastrointestinal adverse effects. There were no significant differences in rates of other adverse effects or additional therapies between IMRT and proton therapy.

"Proton therapy is a high-profile, high-cost prostate cancer treatment. Since 2007, multiple proton facilities have been built, and direct-to-consumer advertising is likely to lead to a substantial increase in use," the authors write. "Overall, our results do not clearly demonstrate a clinical benefit to support the recent increase in proton therapy use for prostate cancer."

The researchers add that the findings that patients receiving IMRT were less likely than those receiving conformal radiation therapy to undergo additional cancer treatments is consistent with the use of IMRT to deliver dose-escalated treatment, resulting in improved cancer control, as demonstrated by randomized trials. "Taken together, these results suggest that IMRT facilitated radiation dose escalation without compromising acceptable long-term morbidity."

"Comparative effectiveness research in localized prostate cancer treatments is needed because of the large number of men with this disease and the continued trend of a rapid increase in use of newer and costlier treatments with unproven clinical benefit," the authors write.

Surgery

Surgery ranks as the most cost-effective type of treatment

The most comprehensive retrospective study ever conducted comparing how the major types of prostate cancer treatments stack up to each other in terms of saving lives and cost effectiveness is reported this week by a team of researchers at the University of California, San Francisco (UCSF).

Appearing in the *British Journal of Urology International,* the work analyzed 232 papers published in the last decade that report results from clinical studies following patients with low-, intermediate- and high-risk forms of prostate cancer who were treated with one or more of the standard treatments – radiation therapy, surgery, hormone therapies and brachytherapy.

The analysis shows that for people with low-risk prostate cancer, the various forms of treatment vary only slightly in terms of survival – the odds of which are quite good for men with this type of cancer, with a 5-year cancer-specific survival rate of nearly 100 percent. But the cost of radiation therapy is significantly more expensive than surgery for low-risk prostate cancer, they found.

For intermediate- and high-risk cancers, both survival and cost generally favored surgery over other forms of treatment – although combination external-beam radiation and brachytherapy together were comparable in terms of quality of life-adjusted survival for high-risk prostate cancer.

"Our findings support a greater role for surgery for high-risk disease than we have generally seen it used in most practice settings," said urologist Matthew Cooperberg, MD, MPH who led the research. Cooperberg is an assistant professor of urology and epidemiology and biostatistics in the UCSF Helen Diller Family Comprehensive Cancer Center.

The UCSF Helen Diller Family Comprehensive Cancer Center is one of the country's leading research and clinical care centers, and it is the only comprehensive cancer center in the San Francisco Bay Area.

Many Treatment Options, but Few Cost Analyses

Localized prostate cancer accounts for about 81 percent of the quarter-million cases of prostate cancers that occur in the United States every year, according to the National Cancer Institute. It is defined by tumors that have not metastasized and spread outside the prostate gland to other parts of the body.

There are multiple types of treatment for this form of the disease, including various types of surgery (open, laparoscopic or robot-assisted); radiation therapy (dose-escalated three-dimensional conformal radiation therapy, intensity-modulated radiation therapy and brachytherapy); hormone therapies; and combinations of each of these. Many men with low-risk prostate cancer do not need any of these treatments, and can be safely observed, at least initially.

Treatment plans for localized prostate cancer often vary dramatically from one treatment center to another. As Cooperberg put it, one person may have surgery, while someone across town with a very similar tumor may have radiation therapy, and a third may undergo active surveillance. All treatment regimens may do equally well.

"There is very little solid evidence that one [approach] is better than another," said Cooperberg. The motivation for the new study, however, was that there are also few data examining the differences in terms of cost-effectiveness – the price to the health care system for every year of life gained, with adjustment for complications and side effects of treatments.

The new study was the most comprehensive cost analysis ever, and it compared the costs and outcomes associated with the various types of treatment for all forms of the disease, which ranged from $19,901 for robot-assisted prostatectomy to treat low-risk disease, to $50,276 for combined radiation therapy for high-risk disease.

The study did not consider two other approaches for dealing with prostate cancer: active surveillance, where patients with low-risk cancer are followed closely with blood tests and biopsies and avoid any initial treatment;

and proton therapy, which is much more expensive and has already been shown in multiple studies not to be cost-effective, said Cooperberg.

Surgery may trump a "watch-and-wait" approach when it comes to treating prostate cancer, especially in younger patients

Surgery may trump a "watch-and-wait" approach when it comes to treating prostate cancer, especially in younger patients, according to a new study.

Death and the spread of cancer were less likely for men who underwent a radical prostatectomy to remove the prostate gland compared to those who didn't -- regardless of age, said study co-author Jennifer Rider, an assistant professor in the department of epidemiology at the Harvard School of Public Health.

"And when we looked at subgroups of age, we found the benefit really appeared to be limited to men with the longest life expectancy," she said.

For years, experts have debated how best to treat the disease -- either using a watch-and-wait approach or removing the gland to help reduce the cancer's spread and extend life.

Dr. Jim Hu, director of robotic and minimally invasive surgery in the urology department of the University of California, Los Angeles, said: "There has been considerable controversy in the United States about PSA [prostate specific antigen] screening for prostate cancer and treatment of prostate cancer."

Experts opposed to surgery say many tumors won't become life-threatening and can be monitored with tests from time to time.

The prostate is a small, walnut-shaped gland that sits below a man's bladder. It produces the fluid that nourishes and transports sperm. According to the American Cancer Association, about 233,000 men in the United States will be diagnosed this year with prostate cancer, which can be detected by a PSA test and by a physical exam.

The Harvard researchers, along with colleagues from Uppsala University Hospital in Sweden, used data from a large Scandinavian prostate cancer study to evaluate about 700 men with early prostate cancer to learn more about life expectancy with the disease.

The men were randomly assigned to either surgery or a watchful-waiting group that received no initial treatment. All were under age 75 and had a life expectancy of 10 or more years. The scientists followed them for up to 23 years, through 2012.

The researchers reported in the March 6 issue of the Journal of the American Medical Association that about 58 percent of the men in the surgery group and 71 percent of the men in the watchful-waiting group died during the study. Prostate cancer was the cause of 18 percent of deaths in the surgery group and about 28 percent in the watchful-waiting group.

Rider said it's important to note that the men in the study had not had their prostate cancer detected using a PSA test and that the data was collected between 1989 and 1999, when the primary form of detection involved a manual exam by the doctor.

"We know PSA screening advances a man's diagnosis by about five to 10 years," Rider said. "So a man today would have the disease diagnosed earlier in his life than in our study."

Hu said it's also key to keep in mind that prostate cancer is typically a slow-growing tumor.

"A lot of the benefit in treating prostate cancer isn't seen for years," Hu said. This study demonstrates that with a median follow-up of 13.4 years, eight men needed to undergo radical prostatectomy to save one from prostate cancer. That's when they saw the survival benefits for surgery versus watchful waiting. This number will continue to go down with longer follow-up."

Rider also said men over 65 who had surgery were less likely to have their cancer spread. "But we don't know if that translates to a mortality benefit," she said.

It was a nice study design, Hu said. "It shows there is a benefit to treating men with prostate cancer," he said.

But he said the findings differ from another recent study by the U.S. Veteran's Administration hospitals that demonstrated that radical prostatectomy did not appear to have a benefit compared to watchful waiting. He said those results, however, could be because the study involved older participants who had other chronic health problems.

Rider said the study results aren't definitive, but she thinks the findings add important information to the debate.

Men Have Overly Optimistic Expectations About Recovery from Prostate Cancer Surgery

Nearly half of men undergoing surgery for prostate cancer expect better recovery from the side effects of the surgery than they actually attain one year after the operation, a University of Michigan Comprehensive Cancer Center study finds.

In addition, prior to surgery, a small proportion of men had expected to have better urinary continence and sexual functions a year after the surgery than they had before it – the exact opposite of what typically happens.

"This is a belief that does not reflect preoperative counseling which, on the contrary, alerts men to urinary and sexual problems after surgery," says study author

Daniela Wittmann, M.S.W, sexual health coordinator at the U-M prostate cancer survivorship program.

The study, published in the August, 2011 issue of the *Journal of Urology*, surveyed 152 men undergoing radical prostatectomy, an operation to remove the prostate. All of the men filled out questionnaires before surgery, after receiving preoperative counseling. The questions asked the men about their expectations of urinary, bowel, hormonal and sexual function a year after the surgery.

The study showed that for the most part, men's expectations of hormonal and bowel function matched what happened one year after surgery. But, when it came to urinary incontinence only 36 percent of the men's expectations corresponded to what happened one year post-surgery.

In addition, only 40 percent of men found what they expected for sexual function to be true one year post-surgery.

Also, 46 percent of the men found worse than expected outcomes in urinary incontinence and 44 percent of men found worse than expected outcomes in sexual function one year after surgery.

"When we provide preoperative education, we can only inform men in terms of overall statistics. We can't predict for the individual," explains Wittmann. "This may mean that, if in doubt, people tend toward being hopeful and optimistic, perhaps overly optimistic."

The researchers suggest that it is important to provide men with tools for urinary and sexual recovery after surgery and with support that will lead to the best possible outcome.

Patients who undergo surgery for prostate cancer at U-M participate in the prostate cancer survivorship program. The program includes partners as well. It is designed to provide men with excellent surgical care along with tailored, couples-oriented support both before and after surgery to help ease recovery from the side-effects of surgery.
"Although preoperative education is very important and should be explicit about the general expectations regarding outcomes, we also need to help men and their partners with the recovery process after surgery in order to help them regain their intimate lives," says Wittmann.

Pain drugs used in prostate gland removal linked to cancer outcome

The methods used to anesthetize prostate cancer patients and control pain when their prostate glands are surgically removed for adenocarcinoma may affect their long-term cancer outcomes, a study led by Mayo Clinic has found. Opioids, painkillers commonly given during and after surgery, may suppress the immune system's ability to fight cancer cells. The research suggests that supplementing general anesthesia with a spinal or epidural painkiller before a radical prostatectomy reduces a patient's need for opioids after surgery, and this finding was associated with a lower risk of cancer recurrence. The findings are published online in the British Journal of Anaesthesia.

The immune system's strength is especially important in cancer surgery because surgical manipulation of a tumor may spread cancer cells. The immune system can be impaired by general anesthesia, the overall stress surgery places on the body and by post-surgical systemic opioid use. The study found better outcomes in radical prostatectomy patients who had general anesthesia supplemented with spinal or epidural delivery of a long-acting opioid such as morphine, than in those who received general anesthesia only.

"We found a significant association between this opioid-sparing technique, reduced progression of the prostate tumor and overall mortality," says senior author Juraj Sprung, M.D., Ph.D., a Mayo Clinic anesthesiologist.

Researchers used Mayo Clinic's prostatectomy registry, anesthesia database and electronic medical records to identify patients who had prostate gland surgery for adenocarcinoma from January 1991 through December 2005. Reports of recurrence of cancer, cancer spread and death were confirmed with patients' physicians.

While promising, the findings must be tested in randomized trials, Dr. Sprung says: "Provided future studies confirm what we've found in this study, maybe down the line this would be a standard of care for pain management in patients undergoing cancer surgery."

Surgery Is Superior to Radiotherapy in Men With Localized Prostate Cancer

Surgery offers better survival benefit for men with localised prostate cancer, according to a large observational study, conducted by a group of researchers in Sweden and the Netherlands.

"The current gold standard management of localised prostate cancer is radical therapy, either as surgery or radiation therapy. This study suggests that surgery is likely superior to radiation for the majority of men who have localized prostate cancer, especially the younger age group and those with no or few comorbidities," said Dr. Prasanna Sooriakumaran, lead study author, of the Karolinska University Hospital in Stockholm.

In their study, Sooriakumaran and colleagues compared the oncologic effectiveness of radical prostatectomy and radiotherapy in prostate cancer, and analysed the mortality outcomes in 34,515 patients treated with up to 15 years follow-up.

Data from Sweden's National Prostate Cancer Registry showed that the men were treated for prostate cancer throughout Sweden with either surgery (n=21,533) or radiotherapy (n=12,982) as their first treatment option and form the study cohort. Patients were categorised by risk group (localised- low risk, localised- intermediate risk, localised- high risk, and non-localized- any T3-4, N+, M+, PSA>50), age (<65, 65-74, ≥75), and Charlson co-morbidity index or CCI (0, 1, ≥2).

In their results, the researchers said radiotherapy patients generally had higher Gleason sums and clinical stages, were older, and had higher PSA than patients that underwent surgery ($p<0.0001$ for all comparisons). Prostate-cancer-mortality (PCM) became a larger proportion of overall mortality as risk group increased for both the surgery and radiotherapy cohorts. The study also showed that for localised prostate cancer patients (risk groups 1-3) survival outcomes favored surgery, and for locally advanced/metastatic patients treatment results were similar.

"This study may herald an increasing use of surgery over radiation in this group. Also, our study concluded that for men with advanced prostate cancer, both modalities appear equivalent and thus the conventional view that surgery is not indicated in this group may be incorrect," explained Sooriakumaran. He added that with their results majority of men with low risk prostate cancer do not die of the disease.

"A very long follow up period is needed to make any comments regarding comparative oncologic outcomes between treatments. Hence, the use of active surveillance may be appropriate in men with low risk disease," Sooriakumaran pointed out.

However, men with intermediate and high-risk disease are at relatively high probability to die from prostate cancer. "Especially when we look at the absolute numbers involved," he said, adding that radical treatment, preferably in the form of surgery, is warranted if possible.

Robot Assisted Prostate Cancer Surgery Compares Favorably

Outcomes from use of a robot to assist surgeons in removal of a cancerous prostate are at least as good, if not better, than the other two techniques used for a radical prostatectomy -- open or laparoscopic surgery -- according to a large meta analysis led by researchers at NewYork-Presbyterian/Weill Cornell.

The study, published February 24 online in European Urology, should help resolve some of the controversy regarding use of the robotic option, known as robot assisted laparoscopic radical prostatectomy (RALP), says the study's lead author, Dr. Ashutosh Tewari, director of the Lefrak Center for Robotic Surgery and director of the Prostate Cancer Institute at New York-Presbyterian Hospital/Weill Cornell Medical Center.

"There is a lot of debate about the best way to remove a cancerous prostate gland," says Dr. Tewari, who is also the Ronald P. Lynch Professor of Urologic Oncology and professor of urology and public health at Weill Cornell Medical College. "Since the robotic technology is expensive, the patient benefits often get intertwined with the societal costs. It is clear, however, that robotic surgery is the most popular surgical modality today. This study represents the largest ever systematic review of patient outcomes comparing robotic-assisted, laparoscopic and open radical prostatectomy.

By analyzing 400 original research articles -- all that have been published to date on the three methods -- Dr. Tewari and his colleagues concluded that RALP is more effective than a pure laparoscopic approach and comparable to an open surgical approach in completely removing cancer from the body. Positive surgical margins, a measure of oncological efficacy, were lower in patients receiving robotic radical prostatectomy as compared to those undergoing laparoscopic prostatectomy.

The researchers also found that robot assisted surgery had fewer intraoperative and perioperative complication rates when compared to both laparoscopic and open approaches. In addition, robotic showed both less intraoperative blood loss and less blood transfusions as compared to open surgery.

The meta analysis included treatment information on 286,876 patients, representing the largest compilation of radical prostatectomy patients to date.

"Understanding the best method to remove the prostate matters," Dr. Tewari says, "because prostate cancer is the most common diagnosed cancer and the second most common cause of cancer death for men in developed countries."

But given the nature of the study, Dr. Tewari says he cannot recommend one surgical approach over another. He emphasizes that surgical approaches need to be adjusted for the technique and experience of the surgeon. Many studies have shown that surgical experience is an independent predictor for outcomes, far beyond the approach alone.

"This paper is innovative in its attempt to unpack the outcomes data, in a systematic way, surrounding the three surgical modalities for prostate cancer treatment, but the data we used were not standardized -- outcome measures differed between studies," he says. "Still I believe the results are meaningful in that it shows RALP has at least as good outcomes as the other methods."

Challenges of Randomized Studies for Prostate Surgery

The three forms of surgery studied are "open radical" in which the prostate is removed via an abdominal incision in the belly button or pubic bone; laparoscopic prostatectomy that requires several small minimally invasive "keyhole" incisions in the abdomen, and robotic surgery, which is a form of laparoscopic surgery. RALP is done through keyholes with the aid of robotic arms that eliminate hand tremor as well as advanced optics that magnify the prostate and surrounding nerves in three-dimensions.

"It is hard to accrue patients for randomized studies. We have an ongoing study open at our institution, investigating the quality of life differences between robotic and open radical prostatectomy. This is designed as a randomized controlled study," he says. "But no one has enrolled because they did not want to be randomized to a treatment they don't prefer. Patients often come, especially to prostate cancer specialists, self-selecting for a particular treatment modality."

So Dr. Tewari and Peter Wiklund, M.D., of Sweden's Karolinska University Hospital, developed a study that examined all of the peer-reviewed studies published on any of the three techniques.

This ambitious effort was aimed at understanding the short-term (30 day) outcomes of the three surgical techniques. Given the short time frame, the meta analysis did not compare outcomes for urinary continence or sexual potency.

The researchers determined that complications and mortality were low for all three methods, suggesting that radical prostatectomy is a safe procedure.

Significant differences found were in the lower positive surgical margin (PSM) rates for RALP compared with laparoscopic surgery and lower intra operative and perioperative complications for RALP in comparison to other modalities. "PSM rates are important because they represent the effectiveness by which cancer is removed," Dr. Tewari says. "The RALP PSM rate was as good as open surgery," he adds.

The researchers also found that both laparoscopic and robotic surgery patients experienced lower rates of blood loss and transfusions and a shorter hospital stay compared with patients who had traditional surgery. Other measures, such as rates of readmission, reoperation, and complications, seemed to favor RALP, the researchers say.

"We would love to be able to directly compare the three prostatectomy surgical techniques, but that may not happen," Dr. Tewari says. "This study is the first to provide an important -- and much needed -- analysis of the short term benefits and risks between curative surgeries that many men rely on."

Study: Robot-assisted surgery for prostate cancer controls the disease for 10 years

Robot-assisted surgery to remove cancerous prostate glands is effective in controlling the disease for 10 years, according to a new study led by researchers at Henry Ford Hospital.

The study also suggested that traditional methods of measuring the severity and possible spread of the cancer together with molecular techniques might, with further research, help to create personalized, cost-effective treatment regimens for prostate cancer patients who undergo the surgical procedure.

The findings apply to men whose cancer has not spread beyond the prostate, and the results are comparable to the well-established and more invasive open surgery to remove the entire diseased prostate and some surrounding tissue.

The research study is published this month online in *European Urology*, the official journal of the European Association of Urology.

"Until our analysis, there was little available information on the long-term oncologic outcomes for patients who undergo robot-assisted radical prostatectomy, or RARP," says Mireya Diaz, Ph.D., Director of Biostatistics at the Henry Ford's Vattikuti Urology Institute (VUI) and lead author of the study.

"As one of the very first hospitals to establish a structured RARP program a little over a decade ago, we were able to determine the long-term effectiveness of the technique thanks to the continued feedback of our patients and the follow-up efforts of the VUI team," Dr. Diaz adds.

The researchers followed 483 consecutive men who had cancer that had not spread outside the prostate and received RARP as their first treatment. All cases were from 2001 to 2003, the earliest years of Henry Ford's robot-assisted prostate surgery program.

Using several standard measures of cancer-treatment success – including biochemical markers of recurrence, incidence of metastasis or the spread of cancer beyond the prostate, and cancer-specific survival – the researchers found that 98.8 percent of the patients survived cancer for 10 years after their surgery.

Further analysis showed that the severity of the cancer after RARP was the best predictor of a recurrence, and the level of prostate-specific antigen, or PSA, in the bloodstream – which is now routinely measured as a test for the possible presence of prostate cancer – can be combined with severity to determine future treatment.

"Disease severity and postoperative PSA measurements can guide physicians in identifying the varying levels of cancer recurrence risk," Dr. Diaz explains. "This includes those patients who can best benefit from secondary treatment as well as long-term monitoring."

The study suggests that persistent PSA levels after RARP signals the risk that cancer may progress and soon require a second or salvage treatment of another kind. Lower risk patients after RARP warrant careful monitoring within five years after surgery and more protracted later, while those at higher risk may need follow-up monitoring beyond 10 years.

Cryoablation (Freezing)

Focal therapy for prostate cancer, in which only the tumor tissue is treated with cryoablation (freezing), can prolong life, result in less complications such as incontinence, and improve post-treatment quality of life. But the long-term effectiveness of focal treatments has not been well-studied. A new analysis that followed patients treated with optimized cryoablation of prostate cancer for an average of 10 years post-treatment is published in Journal of Men's Health, a peer-reviewed publication from Mary Ann Liebert, Inc., publishers. The article is available free on the Journal of Men's Health website.

In the article "Long-Term Results Of Optimized Focal Therapy Of Prostate Cancer: Average 10-Year Follow-Up in 70 Patients," Gary Onik, MD, Carnegie Mellon University (Fort Lauderdale, FL), and coauthors found that long-term cancer control with focal cryoablation therapy was superior to radical whole gland treatments in patients at medium or high risk for disease-free survival.

Prostate Cancer Survivorship

Guidelines Address Long-Term Needs of Prostate Cancer Survivors

Recommendations to Support Primary Care of Estimated 2.8 Million Men with History of Prostate Cancer in the U.S.

New American Cancer Society Prostate Cancer Survivorship Care guidelines released June 10, 2014 outline posttreatment clinical follow-up care for the myriad of long-term and late effects an estimated 2.8 million prostate cancer survivors in the United States may face. The guidelines report is published Early Online in the Society's journal, *CA: A Cancer Journal for Clinicians.*

The guidelines are designed to promote optimal health and quality of life for the posttreatment prostate cancer survivor by facilitating the delivery of comprehensive posttreatment care by primary care clinicians. They are based on recommendations set forth by an expert panel convened as part of the work of the National Cancer Survivorship Resource Center, a collaboration between the American Cancer Society and The George Washington University Cancer Institute, funded by a 5-year cooperative agreement from the Centers for Disease Control and Prevention (CDC).

Prostate cancer survivors represent more than four in ten male cancer survivors and one in five of all cancer survivors in the United States. While guidelines exist for treatment and surveillance for recurrent disease, availability of guidelines for long-term posttreatment care is limited. The American Cancer Society Prostate Cancer Survivorship Care guidelines were developed using a combined approach of evidence synthesis and expert consensus. They address health promotion, surveillance for recurrence and screening for second primary cancers, and the assessment and management of physical and psychosocial long-term and late effects resulting from prostate cancer and its treatment. A key challenge to the development of the guidelines was the limited availability of published evidence informing the clinical management of prostate cancer survivors after treatment.

Among the recommendations:

   * Since information needs evolve as patients transition from treatment through various stages of survivorship, survivor and caregiver information needs should be assessed regularly, with information and support services provided or referred to as necessary.
   * Primary care clinicians should provide regular evaluations of survivors to determine appropriate levels of participation in health promotion and lifestyle modification programs.
   * Primary care clinicians should conduct routine assessments of body mass index among survivors across the prostate cancer survivorship continuum, with

recommendations for limiting consumption of high-calorie foods and beverages for survivors who are overweight or obese.

* Primary care clinicians should educate survivors regarding the association between physical activity and lower overall and prostate cancer-specific mortality and improved quality of life.

* Since smoking after treatment of prostate cancer increases the risk of cancer recurrence and second cancers, primary care clinicians should assess for tobacco use and offer or refer survivors to cessation counseling and resources.

* While existing evidence is not definitive with regard to frequency of monitoring for recurrence using PSA testing, a leading clinical practice guideline, The NCCN guidelines for prostate cancer treatment recommend measuring serum PSA levels every 6 to 12 months for the first 5 years after definitive treatment, and then to recheck annually.

* Clinicians should be aware of a small increased risk of second primary cancers after radiation therapy compared with men receiving surgery. While evidence does not support increased frequency or intensity of screening, adherence to routine ACS screening guidelines for the early detection of any new cancers is recommended.

* Survivors should be assessed for physical (e.g.: urinary, sexual, bowel) and psychosocial effects of prostate cancer and its treatment; the focus of assessment should be tailored to the type of cancer treatment received and current disease state to trigger appropriate self-management and clinical management strategies for

support and therapy.

* Estimates indicate that as many as 30% of patients with prostate cancer experience clinically relevant general distress, 25% have increased anxiety, and nearly 10% experience major depressive disorder. These guidelines affirm early identification, treatment, and ongoing assessment for psychological distress as important aspects of prostate cancer survivorship care.

"We are hopeful that the hard work that went into the development of these much-needed guidelines will pay off in improved care for the approximately 240,000 men diagnosed with prostate cancer every year," said Rebecca Cowens-Alvarado, MPH, principal investigator for the National Cancer Survivorship Resource Center, director of Cancer Control Mission Strategy at the American Cancer Society and co-author of the report. "The adoption of these guidelines will be a critical step forward to improve the delivery of prostate cancer survivorship care."

Last Minute Additions – Latest Research

Depressed men with prostate cancer are diagnosed later stage, get less effective therapies

Depressed men with localized prostate cancer were more likely to be diagnosed with more aggressive prostate cancer, received less effective treatments and survived for shorter times than prostate cancer patients who were not depressed, a UCLA study has found.

The negative outcomes may be the result of several factors such as bias against the mentally ill, depression's impact on biological cancer processes, the depressed man's lack of investment in his general health and disinterest in receiving more effective care, and missed opportunities by physicians to educate patients about prostate cancer screening and treatment, said study lead author Dr. Jim Hu, UCLA's Henry E. Singleton Professor of Urology and director of robotic and minimally invasive surgery at the David Geffen School of Medicine at UCLA.

The population-based observational study using patients from the Surveillance, Epidemiology and End Results (SEER) Medicare database focused on 41,275 men diagnosed with localized prostate cancer between 2004 and 2007 and observed through 2009. Of those, researchers identified 1,894 men with a depressive disorder discovered in the two years before the cancer was diagnosed.

"Men with intermediate- or high-risk prostate cancer and a recent diagnosis of depression are less likely to undergo definitive treatment and experience worse overall survival," Hu said. "The effect of depressive disorders on prostate cancer treatment and survivorship warrants further study, because both conditions are relatively common in men in the United States."

The study appears this week in the early online edition of the Journal of Clinical Oncology, a peer-reviewed journal of the American Society of Clinical Oncology.

Hu said that although demographic and socioeconomic differences can affect treatment and outcomes in prostate cancer, the effect of mental health disorders has remained unclear. Depression has been associated with increased likelihood of not getting the best treatment, as well as lower overall survival in other cancers, including breast and liver cancers. However, little is known about the relationship between depression and diagnosis, treatment and outcomes in prostate cancer. This study helps shed some light on the issue, but further examination is warranted, Hu said.

The study also found that men with prostate cancer who were older, lower income, who had other medical problems, were white or Hispanic, who were unmarried and those residing in non-metropolitan areas were more likely to be depressed.

In addition, depressed men were less likely to seek out definitive therapy such as surgery or radiation in contrast to prostate cancers who were not depressed.

"This was surprising, because depressed men were more likely to see physicians in the two years prior to prostate cancer diagnosis compared to non-depressed men," Hu said.

Prostate cancer is the most frequently diagnosed cancer in men aside from skin cancer. An estimated 233,000 new cases of prostate cancer will occur in the United States in 2014. Of those, nearly 30,000 men will die.

"These results point toward a newly identified disparity in the management of men with incident prostate cancer," the study states. "Considering the marked prevalence of both prostate cancer and depression, additional efforts are needed to better understand and ameliorate the decreased survival following prostate cancer diagnosis in the depressed male patient.

Vasectomy may increase risk of aggressive prostate cancer

Vasectomy was associated with a small increased risk of prostate cancer, and a stronger risk for advanced or lethal prostate cancer according to a new study from Harvard School of Public Health (HSPH). The researchers found that the association remained even among men who received regular PSA screening, suggesting the increased risk of lethal cancer cannot be explained by diagnostic bias. It is the largest and most comprehensive study to date to look at the link between vasectomy and prostate cancer.

The study appears online July 7, 2014 in *Journal of Clinical Oncology.*

"This study follows our initial publication on vasectomy and prostate cancer in 1993, with 19 additional years of follow-up and tenfold greater number of cases. The results support the hypothesis that vasectomy is associated with an increased risk of advanced or lethal prostate cancer," said co-author Lorelei Mucci, associate professor of epidemiology at HSPH.

Vasectomy is a common form of contraception in the U.S., with about 15% of men having the procedure. Prostate cancer is the second-leading cause of cancer death among U.S. men, so identifying risk factors for lethal prostate cancer is important for public health.

The researchers analyzed data from 49,405 U.S. men in the Health Professionals Follow-up Study, who were followed for up to 24 years from 1986 to 2010. During that time, 6,023 cases of prostate cancer were diagnosed, including 811 lethal cases. One in four of the men in this study reported having a vasectomy.

The results showed a 10% increased risk of prostate cancer overall in men who had a vasectomy. Vasectomy was not significantly associated with risk of low-grade cancer. However, vasectomy was associated with a stronger risk of advanced and lethal prostate cancer, with an increased risk of 20% and 19% respectively. Among men who received regular PSA screening, the relative increase in risk of lethal prostate cancer was 56%. The effect appeared to be stronger among men who had a vasectomy at a younger age.

Prior work on this topic raised concerns that the positive associations could be linked to bias. However, in the present study, the researchers had access to diverse information and could rule out potential biases, including that men who have vasectomies may seek more medical care in general, that they may have a higher rates of PSA screening, or that the association was due possible confounding by sexually transmitted infections.

In this study, 16 in 1,000 men developed lethal prostate cancer during 24 years of follow-up. Although the relative increase in the risk associated with vasectomy was significant, this translates to a relatively small increase in absolute difference in the risk of lethal prostate cancer, say the researchers. "The decision to opt for a vasectomy as a form of birth control is a highly personal one and a man should discuss the risks and benefits with his physician," said co-author Kathryn Wilson, research associate in the Department of Epidemiology at HSPH.

Prostate cancer in young men: More frequent, more aggressive?

The number of younger men diagnosed with prostate cancer has increased nearly 6-fold in the last 20 years, and the disease is more likely to be aggressive in these younger men, according to a new analysis from researchers at the University of Michigan Comprehensive Cancer Center.

Typically, prostate cancer occurs more frequently as men age into their 70s or 80s. Many prostate cancers are slow-growing and many older men diagnosed with early stage prostate cancer will end up dying from causes other than prostate cancer.

But, the researchers found, when prostate cancer strikes at a younger age, it's likely because the tumor is growing quickly.

"Early onset prostate cancer tends to be aggressive, striking down men in the prime of their life. These fast-growing tumors in young men might be entirely missed by screening because the timeframe is short before they start to show clinical symptoms," says Kathleen A. Cooney, M.D., professor of internal medicine and urology at the University of Michigan.

Peter Rich was 59 when he was diagnosed with stage 4 prostate cancer. His PSA was only 9, but the disease had already spread to his ribs, spine and lymph nodes.

"To think of mortality was devastating. It was like any major loss -- shock and numbness," says Rich, who had to retire from his job as a school social worker because of his cancer treatment.

Rich was diagnosed six years ago. Average survival for stage 4 disease is generally less than three years.

"What we both said when we got the diagnosis was, well, that's not acceptable," Rich says of himself and his wife, Carol. "I'm a fighter."

Cooney and Scott Tomlins, M.D., Ph.D., assistant professor of pathology at U-M, are leading a new study supported by the U.S. Department of Defense to look at DNA of both normal and cancerous prostate tissue of men diagnosed with advanced prostate cancer before age 61. They will be looking at whether these younger men are more likely to have inherited genetic mutations. For more information on this study, contact the U-M Cancer AnswerLine at 800-865-1125.

Men with a family history of prostate cancer have a two- to three-times greater chance of being diagnosed with prostate cancer. That risk increases for young men with multiple affected relatives.

Prostate cancer runs in Rich's family. Like Rich, his brother was diagnosed in his 50s, and a cousin and uncle had prostate cancer as well.

The new analysis, which appears in *Nature Reviews: Urology,* found that men with early onset prostate cancer had more genetic variants than men diagnosed with prostate cancer at a later age. The researchers suggest that genetic counseling or increased surveillance in younger men with a family history of prostate cancer may be warranted.

American men have a 16 percent risk of developing prostate cancer in their lifetime, but only a 3 percent lifetime risk of dying from it. The challenge, Cooney says, is understanding which subset of prostate cancers are most likely to be aggressive and deadly.

"The unexpectedly poor prognosis of advanced stage early onset prostate cancer supports the idea that a new clinical subtype might exist in the subset of men with early onset prostate cancer. This subtype is more aggressive and requires more specialty expertise, including genetic sequencing," Cooney says.

Appendix- Bladder Cancer

Increased Risk Of Bladder Cancer

New analysis indicates that risk of bladder cancer from smoking greater than previously reported

An analysis of data that includes nearly 500,000 individuals indicates that the risk of bladder cancer among smokers is higher than reported from previous population data, and that the risk for women smokers is comparable with that of men, according to a study in *JAMA*.

More than 350,000 individuals are diagnosed with bladder cancer per year worldwide, including more than 70,000 per year in the United States. Tobacco smoking is the best established risk factor for bladder cancer in both men and women, with previous studies indicating that current cigarette smoking triples bladder cancer risk relative to never smoking, according to background information in the article. "However, the composition of cigarettes has changed during the past 50 years, leading to a reduction in tar and nicotine concentrations in cigarette smoke, but also to an apparent increase in the concentration of specific carcinogens, including beta-napthylamine, a known bladder carcinogen …," the authors write.

Neal D. Freedman, Ph.D., M.P.H., of the National Cancer Institute, Department of Health and Human Services, Rockville, Md., and colleagues conducted a study to examine the association between tobacco smoking and bladder cancer using data from men (n = 281,394) and women (n = 186,134) in the National Institutes of Health-AARP (NIH-AARP) Diet and Health Study, who completed a lifestyle questionnaire and were followed up between October 1995 and December 2006. Previous studies of smoking and incident bladder cancer were identified by systematic review of the available literature.

During the course of follow-up, 3,896 men and 627 women were newly diagnosed with bladder cancer. Cigarette smoking was a significant risk factor for bladder cancer in both sexes. Relative to never smokers, former and current smokers had increased risk of bladder cancer in both men and women. Analysis of the data indicated that former smokers had a 2.2 times increased risk of bladder cancer and that for current smokers, the risk was about 4 times higher, relative to never smokers. "In contrast, the summary risk estimate for current smoking in 7 previous studies (initiated between 1963 and 1987) was 2.94," the authors write.

Ever smoking explained a similar proportion of bladder cancer in both sexes, with population attributable risks of 50 percent in men and 52 percent in women.

The researchers write that factors that may have strengthened the cigarette smoking-bladder cancer association include changes in the constituents of cigarette smoke (such as increased concentrations of beta-napthylamine), and increased awareness of bladder cancer risk in smokers, which may prompt earlier diagnostic workup.

"These results support the hypothesis that the risk of bladder cancer associated with cigarette smoking has increased with time in the United States, perhaps a reflection of changing cigarette composition. Prevention efforts should continue to focus on reducing the prevalence of cigarette smoking."

Meat, especially if it's well done, may increase risk of bladder cancer

People who eat meat frequently, especially meat that is well done or cooked at high temperatures, may have a higher chance of developing bladder cancer, according to a large study at The University of Texas M. D. Anderson Cancer Center presented at the American Association for Cancer Research 101st Annual Meeting - 2010. This risk appears to increase in people with certain genetic variants.

"It's well known that meat cooked at high temperatures generates heterocyclic amines (HCAs) that can cause cancer," said study presenter Jie Lin, Ph.D., assistant professor in M. D. Anderson's Department of Epidemiology. "We wanted to find out if meat consumption increases the risk of developing bladder cancer and how genetic differences may play a part."

Meat-eating habits examined

According to the American Cancer Society, almost 71,000 new cases of bladder cancer were diagnosed in this country last year, and more than 14,000 people died because of the disease. Men are at much higher risk of developing bladder cancer than women.

HCAs form when muscle meats, such as beef, pork, poultry or fish, are cooked at high temperatures. They are products of interaction between amino acids, which are the foundation of proteins, and the chemical creatine, which is stored in muscles. Past research has identified 17 HCAs that may contribute to cancer.

This study, which took place over 12 years, included 884 M. D. Anderson patients with bladder cancer and 878 people who did not have cancer. They were matched by age, gender and ethnicity.

Using a standardized questionnaire designed by the National Cancer Institute (NCI), researchers gathered information about each participant's dietary habits. They then categorized people into four levels, ranging from lowest to highest red meat intake.

The group with the highest red-meat consumption had almost one-and-a-half times the risk of developing bladder cancer as those who ate little red meat.

Specifically, consumption of beef steaks, pork chops and bacon raised bladder cancer risk significantly. Even chicken and fish - when fried - significantly raised the odds of cancer.

The level of doneness of the meat also had a marked impact. People whose diets included well-done meats were almost twice as likely to develop bladder cancer as those who preferred meats rare.

Further questioning of a subset of 177 people with bladder cancer and 306 people without bladder cancer showed that people with the highest estimated intake of three specific HCAs were more than two-and-a-half times more likely to develop bladder cancer than those with low estimated HCA intake.

"To quantify intakes of HCAs, we began three or four years ago to gather information on meat-cooking methods and doneness level, and then used a program developed by the NCI to estimate intakes of three major HCAs," Lin said. "These data gave important information about the relationship between HCAs and bladder cancer."

Genetic variants increase incidence

To take the investigation a step further, researchers analyzed each participant's DNA to find if it contained genetic variants in the HCA metabolism pathways that may interact with red meat intake to increase the risk of cancer.

People with seven or more unfavorable genotypes as well as high red-meat intake were at almost five times the risk of bladder cancer.

"This research reinforces the relationship between diet and cancer," said Xifeng Wu, M.D., Ph.D., professor in M. D. Anderson's Department of Epidemiology and lead author on the study. "These results strongly support what we suspected: people, who eat a lot of red meat, particularly well-done red meat, such as fried or barbecued, seem to have a higher likelihood of bladder cancer. This effect is compounded if they carry high unfavorable genotypes in the HCA-metabolism pathway."

Wu said this research is a step toward a future in which a comprehensive cancer-risk prediction model will integrate environmental, diet and genetic risk factors to predict an individual's chances of developing cancer.

Red meat increases risk for bladder cancer

Two components of red meat — dietary protein and dietary iron — may combine to form powerful carcinogens, N-nitroso compounds, which increase risk for bladder cancer. Moreover, individuals with reduced ability to reverse the effects of N-nitroso compounds because of a genetic variation in their RAD52 gene could be at particularly high risk.

Chelsea Catsburg, a doctoral student at the Keck School of Medicine of the University of Southern California, Los Angeles, presented these data at the 11th Annual AACR International Conference on Frontiers in Cancer Prevention Research, held here Oct. 16-19, 2012.

Dietary protein is made up of amino acids, which can be naturally metabolized into biogenic amines, according to Catsburg. Research has shown that the processing and storage of meat increases amine concentrations. When these amines are in the presence of nitrites, they generate nitrosamines, which have carcinogenic properties. In addition, heme iron, found in red meat, has been shown to increase the formation of nitrosamines from amines.

"Nitrosamine formation occurs predominantly in the stomach and intestines, so these exposures have been studied extensively in relation to gastric cancer and somewhat in relation to colorectal cancer," Catsburg said. "However, there is evidence that these reactions also take place in the bladder, particularly in the presence of infection."

Catsburg and colleagues had previously found that meat groups with high heme and high amine concentrations, such as salami and liver, increased risk for bladder cancer. In this study, they examined whether genetic variation in DNA repair enzymes, available to correct the damage caused by these endogenously formed carcinogens, modified these associations.

The researchers tested 627 single-nucleotide polymorphisms in 27 genes involved in N-nitroso compound metabolism or DNA repair. They collected data from 355 bladder cancer cases and 409 controls in the Los Angeles Bladder Cancer Study.

"We found that a polymorphism in the RAD52 gene modified the effect of these exposures," Catsburg said. "This polymorphism is suspected to reduce the DNA repair activity of the RAD52 protein, and the association of these meat groups and bladder cancer risk was significantly higher in individuals with one or more copies of this polymorphism."

These results further support recommendations by the World Cancer Research Fund to limit red meat intake and to avoid processed meats to reduce risk for stomach and bowel cancer, according to the researchers.

"This study suggests that these exposures may also affect secondary organs such as the bladder," Catsburg said. "Individuals at risk for bladder cancer may wish to avoid intake of red and processed meats, especially if they have genetic polymorphisms that reduce DNA repair activity and make them more vulnerable to the effects of carcinogens."

Depression increased bladder cancer mortality

As part of an ongoing, large-scale epidemiologic study of bladder cancer, Chen and colleagues collected clinical and mental health information on 464 patients with bladder cancer. They assessed patients' depression levels with the Center for Epidemiologic Studies Depression Scale (CES-D).

Depression symptoms alone affected mortality: Patients with CES-D scores of 16 or greater had a median survival time of 58 months, while those with scores below 16 had a median survival time longer than 200 months. In addition, patients with CES-D scores of 16 or greater had a 1.89-fold increased risk for all-cause mortality compared with patients with CES-D scores less than 16.

In addition, the researchers pointed to evidence that smoking cessation, weight loss and increased physical activity can potentially improve survival.

"In terms of building a prediction model for bladder cancer mortality, current models only focus on clinical variables, such as treatment and tumor stage and grade," Chen said. "Our study suggests that psychological factors and perhaps lifestyle changes could be included in this prediction model."

Fighting Bladder Cancer

Like prostate cancer, bladder cancer patients may benefit from anti-androgen therapy

Bladder cancer patients whose tumors express high levels of the protein CD24 have worse prognoses than patients with lower CD24. A University of Colorado Cancer Center study published today in the Proceedings of the National Academy of Sciences shows that CD24 expression may depend on androgens – and that anti-androgen therapies like those currently used to treat prostate cancer may benefit bladder cancer patients.

Vitamin D + TB Vaccine: Allies in Fight Against Bladder Cancer?

The tuberculosis vaccine is often used as a treatment for bladder cancer, and adding vitamin D might improve the vaccine's effectiveness, according to new research from the University of Rochester Medical Center presented at the American Urological Association annual meeting.

Yi-Fen Lee, Ph.D., associate professor of Urology at URMC, has conducted a pre-clinical study in a mouse model showing that a combination of vitamin D therapy and the Bacillus Calmette-Guerin (BCG) vaccine greatly improves bladder cancer survival. The next phase, an early clinical trial in patients, will begin soon as part of a collaborative research project between the URMC'sJames P. Wilmot Cancer Center and the Roswell Park Cancer Institute in Buffalo.

The connection between vitamin D and tuberculosis was established long ago, when ancient societies sent people with TB into the sunlight for therapy. Increasing vitamin D levels is known to wake up cells and trigger an immune response whenever infection or inflammation is present.

Also well established is the use of the TB vaccine to treat several forms of bladder cancer. The vaccine works by pushing the body's immune system to fight the cancer cells. However, approximately 30 to 40 percent of people with bladder cancer who receive the vaccine do not respond to it.

Lee is investigating whether a lack of vitamin D in these patients might explain the poor response.

Prior studies have shown that BCG, the modified bacteria that causes TB, turns on a toll-like receptor signal that makes more vitamin D receptors and induces a key enzyme that converts to the most potent, bioactive form of vitamin D, or 1,25-hydroxylvitamin D3. So Lee thought it was likely that boosting the levels of vitamin D in the body would activate this process, enhancing the vaccine.

The mouse study involved four arms: a control group, a group that received vitamin D treatment alone, a group that received BCG treatment alone, and a fourth group that received the combination of vitamin D and the BCG vaccine. The latter (combination therapy) group was the only group in which 100 percent survived bladder cancer, Lee said.

"Vitamin D appears to be critical to the success of BCG immunotherapy," Lee said, although she does not advise taking high doses of vitamin D unless under medical supervision. "Just as importantly, though, we have shown the migration and signaling involved in establishing vitamin D as a biomarker that can be easily measured."

Regular exercise may increase the odds of bladder cancer survival

"Bladder cancer is among the top 10 most common cancers in the United States, with an estimated 72,000 new cases occurring each year," Dr. Mirza Moben, an assistant professor of urology at the University of Kansas Medical Center, said in a news release from the American Urological Association.

The study was presented at the May 2014 American Urological Association annual meeting.

The study, from researchers at the University of California, San Diego, involved national survey data on more than 200,000 people. Of these, 48 percent were men, and 73 percent were white. The participants provided information on their level of physical activity and their body mass index -- a measurement that can help determine if someone is a normal weight for their height.

Although the investigators found no link between ethnicity or gender and survival rates for bladder cancer, they did find that exercise may prevent bladder cancer deaths. The participants who exercised were more likely to survive their disease than those who didn't exercise. Even light or moderate exercise might help, the study authors suggested.

A past history of smoking was also linked to a tripled likelihood of dying from bladder cancer compared to those who never smoked, the researchers added.

However, while the study found an association between exercise, smoking and survival rates, it did not prove a cause-and-effect relationship.

Higher Intake of Fruits and Vegetables = Lower Risk of Bladder Cancer

University of Hawaii Cancer Center Researcher Song-Yi Park, PhD, along with her colleagues, recently discovered that a greater consumption of fruits and vegetables may lower the risk of invasive bladder cancer in women.

The investigation was conducted as part of the Multiethnic Cohort (MEC) Study, established in 1993 to assess the relationships among dietary, lifestyle, genetic factors, and cancer risk. Park and her fellow researcher's analyzed data collected from 185,885 older adults over a period of 12.5 years, of which 581 invasive bladder cancer cases were diagnosed (152 women and 429 men).

After adjusting for variables related to cancer risk (age, etc.) the researchers found that women who consumed the most fruits and vegetables had the lowest bladder cancer risk. For instance, women consuming the most yellow-orange vegetables were 52% less likely to have bladder cancer than women consuming the least yellow-orange vegetables. The data also suggested that women with the highest intake of vitamins A, C, and E had the lowest risk of bladder cancer. No associations between fruit and vegetable intake and invasive bladder cancer were found in men.

"Our study supports the fruit and vegetable recommendation for cancer prevention, said Park. "However, further investigation is needed to understand and explain why the reduced cancer risk with higher consumption of fruits and vegetables was confined to only women."

Treatment For Bladder Cancer

Nearly all patients with high-grade bladder cancer do not receive guideline-recommended care

A study at UCLA's Jonsson Comprehensive Cancer Center found that nearly all patients with high-grade, non-invasive bladder cancer are not receiving the guideline-recommended care that would best protect them from recurrence, a finding that researchers characterized as alarming.

In fact, out of the 4,545 bladder cancer patients included in the study, only one received the comprehensive care recommended by the American Urology Association and the National Comprehensive Cancer Network.

Receiving the recommended comprehensive care for high-grade bladder cancer is critical because it can significantly minimize the likelihood that patients will die from their cancer, said Dr. Karim Chamie, a postdoctoral fellow in urologic oncology and health services research and lead author of the study.

"We were surprised by the findings in this study, particularly in an era when many suggest that doctors over-treat patients and do too much in the name of practicing defensive medicine," Chamie said. "This study suggests quite the contrary, that we don't do enough for patients with bladder cancer. If this was a report card on bladder cancer care in America, I'd say we're earning a failing grade."

The study is published July 11, 2011 in the early online edition of *CANCER,* a peer-reviewed journal of the American Cancer Society.

The study then investigated the cause of poor compliance. What they found was that non-compliance knew no boundaries and that patient-level factors such as age, race, ethnicity or socioeconomic status had very little impact. Instead, non-compliance with guideline-recommended care was primarily attributed to urologists. The patients in the study were elderly, but capable of withstanding these simple measures.

"It wasn't their age, race, ZIP code or how wealthy they were. It all came down to who their doctor was," Chamie said

Dr. Mark S. Litwin, professor of urology and public health and senior author of the study, said it's not clear why physicians are not routinely following established guidelines for care.

"It is puzzling, because strong evidence supports those guidelines," Litwin said. "But this is a wake-up call to all physicians caring for patients with bladder cancer. We know definitively what constitutes high-quality care. Now we just need to make sure it happens."

Patients with primary high-grade bladder cancer, which has not yet invaded the muscle of the bladder, have a 50 to 70 percent chance of their cancer coming back in the bladder following treatment. They also have a 30 to 50 percent chance of the cancer becoming more aggressive and invading into the muscle, where it is much harder to treat. Once the cancer invades the muscle, the bladder and surrounding organs must be removed and both the quality and the quantity of the patient's life are significantly impacted, Chamie said.

Chamie said that, at diagnosis, about 75 percent of bladder patients have disease that has not invaded the muscle. So treating those patients with the guideline-recommended care to help minimize recurrences and prevent invasion of the tumor into the muscle could help a large number of patients.

The recommended medical guidelines call for injecting a cancer-killing drug directly into the bladder to minimize recurrence and progression. They also recommend an intense follow-up schedule, including the repeated use of a scope to evaluate the bladder from the inside, a procedure called cystoscopy, and a urine test that is similar to a pap smear every three months to check for abnormal cells.

Only one patient in the study, which analyzed date from Surveillance, Epidemiology and End Results (SEER)-Medicare linked database, was given the recommended care. The study also found that nearly half of urologists treating these patients had not performed at least one cystoscopy, one urine test, and one infusion of the cancer-killing drug into the bladder.

To rectify the situation, Chamie and Litwin suggest a quality-improvement initiative and or changes to physician reimbursements. To complicate matters, despite the poor compliance rate, bladder cancer is the most expensive malignancy to treat on a per-patient level. While improving compliance with changes to physician reimbursement or a quality improvement initiative will increase healthcare costs in the short term, preventing recurrences or progression of the cancer likely will cut costs in the long term.

"We have to improve compliance and there are two ways to do that: Modify our reimbursement schedules to provide incentives to doctors to follow the guidelines, or go out and interact and educate the community urologists - who are delivering the vast majority of bladder cancer care - on the importance of providing compliant care," Chamie said. "Unlike some patients diagnosed with bladder cancer after having it spread to other sites when it's too late to treat effectively, or those with low-grade tumors that are not likely to ever be aggressive, this is a potentially curable cohort of patients. If we don't do a good enough job treating these cancers, we're going to lose these patients."

Improved radical surgery techniques provide positive outcomes for bladder cancer patients

Bladder cancer patients who have radical surgery at university hospitals can benefit from excellent local control of the disease, acceptable clinical outcomes and low death rates, according to research in the urology journal *BJUI*.

Researchers studied 2,287 patients who had radical cystectomy surgery, where the bladder is removed, together with nearby tissue and organs as required. The surgery was performed at eight Canadian academic centres between 1998 and 2008.

The study found that there were three independent factors, apart from pathological stage at surgery, that influenced survival rates. Patients who smoked had lower survival rates, while patients who had pelvic lymphadenectomy - lymph nodes removed from the pelvic area - had higher survival rates, as did patients who received adjuvant chemotherapy, which aims to destroy microscopic cancer cells left after surgery.

However, the researchers found that neoadjuvant chemotherapy - which is often recommended prior to surgery to improve outcomes - tends to be under utilised for bladder cancer in Canada.

"Recent advances in combined radiation with chemotherapy have challenged the role of radical cystectomy (RC) with pelvic lymphadenectomy, which is used to treat muscle invasive and refractory non-muscle invasive bladder cancer" says co-author Dr Wassim Kassouf, from McGill University Health Centre, Quebec, Canada.

"These bladder-preservation strategies are potentially attractive in terms of health-related quality of life and cancer outcomes, but they only tend to work in highly selected patients.

"Advances in RC surgery have improved surgical care and techniques and reduced complications and mortality rates. The aim of our study was to evaluate a contemporary series of patients with bladder cancer to assess the clinical outcomes and identify any variables that affected their long-term health."

Key findings of the study included:

- 79% of the patients were male, the median age was 68 and the average follow-up of live patients was just over 29 months. 66% reported a family history of tobacco smoking.
- More than three-quarters of the patients had high-grade tumours. Pathological specimen examination revealed no evidence of cancer in 7% of patients, muscle invasive disease in 73% and positive nodal involvement in 25%.
- Adjuvant chemotherapy was offered to 19% of patients and neoadjuvant chemotherapy to just over 3%.
- All patients had previously undergone transurethral resection of bladder tumours and the median time from

this to RC surgery was 49 days. This is similar to waiting times reported in international studies conducted in Sweden (49 days), the USA (42 days) and Germany (54 days).
- The 30, 60 and 90-day death rates were 1.3%, 2.6% and 3.2% respectively. Cancer returned in 33% of patients within a median of 10 months. Local recurrence rates were 6% in the overall group and 4% in the organ-confirmed node-negative group.
- The five-year overall, recurrence-free and cancer-specific survival rates were 57%, 48% and 67% respectively.

Multivariate analysis showed that lower pathological stage, negative surgical margins, receipt of adjuvant chemotherapy, performance of pelvic lymphadenectomy and an absence of smoking were associated with prolonged disease-specific and overall survival.

"Our study shows that very good results can be achieved when RC is performed at academic centres within a universal healthcare system and that it remains an effective clinical option for treating patients with bladder cancer" says Dr Kassouf.

Cutting-edge gene therapy for bladder cancer

Bladder cancer, most frequently caused by smoking and exposure to carcinogens in the workplace, is one of the top 10 most common forms of cancer in men and women in the U.S. More than 70 percent of bladder cancers are diagnosed in stage T1 or less and have not invaded the muscle layer. At these early stages, standard treatment is surgery (transurethral resection) and the burning away of tumors with high energy electricity (fulguration). Many patients also may receive subsequent intravesical chemotherapy because there is often a high-risk for cancer recurrence.

The prognosis for recurrent cancer is poor, which drives clinician-scientists like William Larchian, MD, Urologic Oncologist, University Hospitals Urology Institute at University Hospitals Case Medical Center, and Associate Professor of Surgery, Case Western Reserve University School of Medicine, and his colleagues to develop an immunotherapy for bladder cancer that will stimulate the body's own natural defense mechanisms to cure the disease and prevent recurrence.

"What is interesting is that our bodies are capable of identifying, responding to and killing tumor cells naturally," explained Dr. Larchian. "We are developing a vaccination system to enhance this response and drive an effective immune response against existing and future bladder tumor cells in patients diagnosed with bladder cancer."

IL-2, a cytokine-signaling molecule, stimulates the T-cell immune response to cancer cells in the bladder. Dr. Larchian and his colleagues have developed a system that reliably introduces multiple copies of IL-2 DNA into bladder cancer cells.

"This method allows for more gene copies to enter the cells," he said, "and we are able to see higher rates of transfection compared to retroviral methods."

The enhanced IL-2 protein expression has been shown to successfully stimulate T-cell response and eliminate bladder tumors in a mouse model, particularly when followed by transfection with B7.1 gene. The addition of the B7.1 gene, which encodes an immune co-stimulatory molecule, enhanced T-cell production logarithmically and produced a 70 percent cure rate. Rechallenge with new cancer cells was also prevented. Clinical translation of this research has been submitted for Institutional Review Board approval at UH Case Medical Center.

Other research by Dr. Larchian and his colleagues aims to leverage this work to develop a gene-therapy system that can be utilized to deliver other key defense genes.

"Our future pursuits," he said, "will include using this system with very specific biological response modifiers, including anti-angiogenesis factors, and with the tumor suppressor gene, MCP3." Dr. Larchian also is developing a targeted drug delivery system using nanoparticles for bladder cancer treatment.

CPSIA information can be obtained at www.ICGtesting.com
Printed in the USA
LVOW01s0250140115

422748LV00038B/1049/P